I0426775

The
Skip a Day Diet

Copyright © 2008 Dennis Brooks

All Rights Reserved. Cram School

No part of this book may be reproduced, stored in a retrieval system,
or transmitted by any means, electronic, mechanical, photocopying,
recording, or otherwise, without written permission from the author.

ISBN: 1-4196-9234-8
ISBN-13: 9781419692345

Visit www.booksurge.com to order additional copies.

The
Skip a Day Diet

Introducing
Volume Weight Loss

Learn to turn off your appetite!

Dennis Brooks
Beat Obesity Boot Camp

Table of Contents

CHAPTER ONE

Introducing the Skip A Day Diet

THE SKIP A DAY DIET was developed so that dieters would have a way to deliberately target and burn their stored body fat. The concept is simple. The dieter should eat a full healthy meal one day to provide the body with the nourishment it needs. The next day, the dieter should skip eating and force the body to draw on stored fat and use it for energy. With this approach, the dieter will always be only twenty-four hours from a full, healthy meal when dieting every other day.

The diet allows you to consume your full nutritional allowance the first day and eat very little the second day. People, who have a recommended dietary allowance of 2,400 calories per day, may consume 1800 calories on eat-day and 600 calories on diet-day. This will give them 1,200 calories per day for the two-day period.

The main thing that allows the diet to work is appetite control and volume. Also, when you follow the instructions and get a good night's sleep after a day of eating, your appetite will disappear (for the most part) until the next day. Also, you will be able to adjust your meal times so that they are close to your rest time. This will help cut out snacking.

Here is how the diet forces the body to give up its stored fat. The first night of the two-day cycle, your body will process the food you ate that day and store the nutrients in its twenty-hour reserve. The next day your body will distribute the nutrients you consumed the day before. The second night, your body will draw on your stored fat and bring your reserve energy level back up to full. This way you will be deliberately targeting and burning stored body fat, which will lead to a permanent weight loss.

This approach allows you to diet one day at a time and lose weight. Anyone can try the diet for a few days by taking the test. By taking the diet test first, a would-be dieter can determine if the diet will work before spending too much time on it. The Skip A Day Diet is not expensive to use. With this diet, you can use ordinary food until you reach your target weight.

Also, dieting will get much easier after you get started. Then it takes only a few weeks to overcome the physical and mental challenges that come with losing weight. That is no big obstacle because if others can use this diet to lose weight, you can do it too.

The best thing about the diet is that it's free. You pay nothing, and you can stay on it as long as you like. There are no special foods or supplements to buy and no restrictions on the foods you eat. If you are interested in losing weight, take the Skip A Day Diet test. Then give the diet a test drive to see if it's right for you.

CHAPTER TWO

The Skip A Day Test

To TEST THE diet properly, you must go through one complete cycle, which is one day of eating and one day of dieting. It will take forty-eight hours to complete the test. After you pass the test, you can start losing weight on the Skip A Day Diet. The test consists of an eat-day and a diet-day. If you can pass the test, there is a good chance that you can lose weight with the Skip A Day Diet. If you fail the test, chances are you succumbed and ate something or drank something that triggered your appetite.

Try the Skip A Day Diet. Take the Test!

If you would like to try the Skip A Day Diet, get started right away. The test is made up of a set of instructions to be followed over a period of two days. The first day is the eat-day. The second day is the diet-day. You will know if it works within two days, because of this test. After you pass the test, you can start losing weight on the Skip A Day Diet.

First Day, Eat-Day

Breakfast Time:

When you get up in the morning, eat a full-size breakfast and try to avoid eating table sugar or concentrated sweets. If you do not normally eat breakfast, eat what would be equal to a small bowl of cereal with 1 percent or skim milk and a piece of fruit. If you normally eat a large breakfast, do not cut back on the food, but try to limit the fat to about twenty grams. During the test the exact amount of food you have for breakfast is not critical. Other food choices for breakfast include toast, biscuits and gravy, hash browns, pancakes (without syrup), or any combination of those foods. You may substitute equally for items not mentioned here.

Snack Time:

If you need to snack between meals, use cheese, crackers, fruit, and vegetables. Stay away from sweets such as candy, soda, ice cream, cake, or pie. If you do not normally have a snack, skip the snack.

Lunch Time:

A six-inch sub sandwich with a green salad and a glass of water would be ideal for lunch. Since most people eat more than that, the next best thing would be a foot-long sub sandwich with lots of vegetables. Another good lunch choice would be a sandwich with a bowl of soup. It does not have to be a sub sandwich; any sandwich will be sufficient as long as it includes plenty of bread and vegetables. If you do not like sandwiches, go ahead and have a garden salad or chicken salad with rolls or have a vegetable dish. Avoid sugars and sweets.

Dinner Time:

Try to delay eating dinner until about six p.m., although anytime between five and seven p.m. will be good. For dinner, eat a regular meal such as fish, chicken, steak, or chops. Try to keep the meat serving below three ounces and trim the fat. Eat at least two servings of green vegetables: canned, fresh, or frozen. If you normally eat a lot for dinner, have one or two extra slices of bread with your meal and continue to avoid sugar.

Bed Time:

If you are still hungry at bedtime, have bread with cheese or milk and cereal (no sugar). Try to finish eating about ninety minutes before bedtime to prevent an upset stomach. If you have a sweet tooth that's difficult to control, give yourself a treat. Have a small piece of chocolate or something else you like. Go to bed and get a good night's sleep.

CHAPTER THREE

Second Day, Diet-Day

W HEN YOU GET up in the morning, eat absolute nothing because you will not be hungry. Have your favorite beverage for breakfast while reading the paper or doing whatever you do in the morning. Keep your meal restricted to coffee, tea, or water. Use no sweetener at all in your drinks, if possible. However, if you just have to have something sweet, use an artificial sweetener. Finish your beverage and go to work, either in the home or outside the home. Drink water throughout the day whenever you get thirsty. The amount of water you drink may depend on your activity level.

All of the nourishment you consumed the day before will be still with you in the morning when you wake up. During the night your body will have balanced your energy level and shut off your appetite. You should be able to go all day without eating.

However, if your appetite is so strong that you just have to eat something, first delay eating as long as you can. Then have up to 600 calories in healthy snacks such as cheese and bread, toast and jam, or soup and salad. Then try to go to bed and get a good night's sleep. If you consumed more than the 600 calories, you failed the test. Try it again another time.

If you ate nothing at all before bedtime or kept the calorie count low, you are almost there. Also, if you can get up in the morning and **not** rush into the kitchen and eat breakfast right away, you have made it. You're in! Congratulations and welcome to the "Skip A Day Diet Club."

If you followed the instructions to the letter except for eating only the food necessary to take medicine, you are a good candidate for the Skip A Day Diet. Before you learn to use, refine, and adjust the diet to suit your specific needs, read the following overview to understand what happened during the two-day test period.

TEST RESULTS (OVERVIEW)

During the first day, you ate enough food to provide your body with a full, balanced nutritional allowance. You had the correct ratio of protein, carbohydrates, vitamins, and minerals. As you filled your stomach by eating the three meals, your body processed some of the food to provide energy for that day. At bedtime your stomach was still full.

While you were sleeping, your body processed the rest of the food and stored the nutritional content, so that it would be distributed to different areas based on the needs of your organs and muscles. It also prepared other reserve nourishment needed for the next day's activities. If some important nutrient was missing from your meals, the body made it and stored it along with the carbohydrates, fat, and protein.

If you did not eat enough fat for the next day's activities, the body drew on its stored fat and placed it into the reserve so that it would be available for the next day, which was diet day. This brought your twenty-four-hour reserve energy level up to full. The balanced meals you consumed the day before and the fat released into your system during the night was enough to give you another full day's reserve. Nutritionally, you were still full the next morning when you woke up on diet-day.

All the food you ate the day before was enough to allow you to skip a day and take you through the diet period. You only needed to drink water. There was no need to eat again until your food reserve ran low during the third day.

Now that you know how the Skip A Day Diet works, you need to learn how food interacts in the body while providing nourishment. To build a more efficient weight loss program, learn how to use this diet with different foods, exercises, and other activities that will allow you to lose weight faster.

The rest of the book explains nutrition and exercise relative to the Skip A Day Diet. It also explains the volume concept and suggests basic meal plans to help you lose weight faster. When you master the Skip A Day Diet, you will be able to lose weight at a slow, constant rate. To improve your health, study the material on exercise and nutrition. It will help you understand how the Skip A Day Diet and exercise can work together to help you lose weight.

CHAPTER FOUR

Continuing the Skip A Day Diet After the Test

A FTER THE TEST period, start to reduce the number of times you eat each day by cutting out breakfast. Hold out until 11:30 a.m. or 12 p.m. before eating lunch by drinking water until you break the breakfast habit. You can eat just about anything you want on the eat-day. However, have only a small lunch. Eventually you will be able to skip lunch altogether.

The second diet-day might be more difficult to manage because your habitual appetite will be stronger at meal times. Before the first diet-day, you will have eaten two days in a row before dieting. Before the second diet-day, you will have eaten only one day before dieting. Make sure you have enough nourishment by eating enough on eat-day so that your body will not run out of energy on diet-day. It takes a while for your body to learn to draw on and use its stored fat.

Keep in mind that if you eat anything on diet day, it could trigger your appetite and cause you to start eating. If you get really hungry on diet-day, hold out as long as you can and stay busy. Usually the hunger will pass after a while. If necessary, have a cup of soup with bread in the afternoon and try to hold out the rest of the day without eating. Also, if you cannot hold out until the next morning because of your habitual appetite, have light snacks such as bread with some type of spread. Your late night snack may include an egg sandwich instead of junk food. In every case, try to keep the calorie count below 600 on diet-day.

Always try to hold off as much as possible and go to bed without eating much on diet day because it's too easy to just eat what you want, when you want it. Remind yourself that you are dieting and must not eat every time you feel like it. If you do have snacks on diet-day, choose foods that are filling rather that those that taste great.

Take a break from the diet once or twice a month only if necessary. Otherwise, continue to lose weight until you reach your goal. It will get easier as time goes by.

CHAPTER FIVE

Appetite Control, What We're Up Against

I N ORDER TO develop a plan for appetite control, you need to learn as much as you can about the appetite, which is a complex system that involves the senses, chemical processes in the body, and the psychological makeup of the human mind. Also, all of our senses can play a part in activating our appetite in one way or another. The senses, taste, smell, sight, touch, and hearing can all be used to remind us that it's time to eat.

Psychology or common sense is the reasoning that says we must eat regularly to live and remain healthy, but there is more to it than that. When the appetite is triggered, the body releases different chemicals into the stomach and brain to tell us when to eat and when to stop eating. Our need to eat, to stay alive along with our appetite, make it difficult to skip a meal knowing that our health and well being depends on good food.

Then there is our metabolism, which is the process of using food for energy, growth, development, and maintenance over a lifetime. Trying to understand either appetite or metabolism is difficult at the least. However, trying to learn how they're all associated with each other and how they interact is even more of a challenge.

Nevertheless, we are beginning to understand more and more of what's happening through the science of appetite control and weight loss. New research is helping us understand the cause of excess weight gain and is helping us come up with ways to help turn it around. However, getting people motivated enough to try and stay on a new weight loss program is another challenge.

By gathering and studying facts regarding the science of appetite, we can see bits and pieces of the picture gradually developing. We can use the facts to help us make assumptions, deductions, and educated guesses about appetite control and food choices. Also, the facts can help us formulate a plan for action for solving the problems we are facing. Let's study one of the important facts about the appetite.

Since we know from research and experience that it takes about twenty minutes for the appetite to go away after the stomach is full, we can assume that people are programmed to overeat. We can also assume that at one time in the past, it was okay to overeat because of the programming. Now that food is plentiful, and we have evolved pass the stage where it is necessary to over eat, what can we do?

Let's start by studying the chemical reactions that make us hungry enough to overeat in the first place. In 1999 a hormone called ghrelin, which is often referred to as the hunger hormone because it causes hunger, was identified. The body releases ghrelin into the stomach each day during the times we normally eat our regular meals. This causes an empty feeling in the stomach, which lets us know it's time to eat.

When ghrelin reaches the brain, it goes to three areas: the hindbrain, which controls the body's automatic, unconscious processes; the hypothalamus, which governs metabolism; and the mesolimbic reward center in the midbrain, where feelings of pleasure and satisfaction are processed. This powerful series of events guarantees that when ghrelin is released into the system, you will respond by eating something if food is available.

As scientists continue to study ghrelin, they are finding out more about how it works in the body. They have found that the levels of ghrelin spike at mealtimes. The release of ghrelin into the stomach keeps pace with your feeding schedule. That's why we get hungry three times a day whether our bodies need the food or not. Also, whenever there is a change in the mealtime pattern, there is a change in the times when ghrelin spikes in the stomach. Even without the spikes, there are low levels of ghrelin in our stomach at all times of the day, which accounts for our need to have two or three snacks in between meals.

Another chemical found in the stomach is called cholecystokinin or (CCK). It is a peptide that is released by the upper intestine. It then travels to the brain to give you a feeling of satisfaction so that you will stop eating when you get full. However, the effect of CCK is temporary. That is why you may get hungry after returning home from having an expensive meal at a nice restaurant.

Even CCK is limited in its ability to prevent weight gain. CCK does no good if the person consumes a nutrient rich meal that consists of mostly fats and sugars in foods such as fried chicken, white rice, white bread, cookies, and milkshakes because a high calorie meal such as that can contain about 3,000 calories or more. Also, after the stomach gets full, it could be another twenty minutes before CCK is released into the intestine to signal that the stomach is full. If your stomach gets full before CCK reaches the brain, you may continue to eat. This causes the stomach to stretch, which allows the person to consume extra food.

Next in line are two other hormones to stop us from eating: GLP-1 and PYY. They are used to make sure you stop eating before you overeat. They are also produced in the stomach and travels to the brain. From the brain, they send out signals to let you know that you have had enough to eat. They also tell your stomach to stop processing food so that nothing else goes into the lower intestines. This gives the stomach time to digest and process some of the food you have eaten. Also, GLP-1 adjusts blood chemistry by stimulating the pancreas to release more insulin. The insulin helps to store all of the excess sugar into the body's fat cells. This process should regulate the amount of food you eat and help keep you healthy by eliminating sugar from the bloodstream. However, this system seems to eventually fail because of a heavy sugar overload.

Another appetite-suppressing hormone was discovered in 1994, called leptin. It is supposed to cause people, who are overweight, to eat less. If it worked the way it should, fat people would eat less than skinny people. A person's body fat produces this hormone, and it is usually produced in direct proportion to the amount of fat tissue the person has. The fatter you are, the more leptin your fat cells produce. Once in the bloodstream, it travels to the hypothalamus, which is one of the same regions of the brain targeted by ghrelin. When it reaches the hypothalamus, it muffles the signals caused by the ghrelin that stimulated the appetite in the first place.

The discovery of leptin caused excitement in the world of dieting. Researchers thought that obese people were simply suffering from a shortage of leptin in the body. It would be simple to supplement the hormone and watch the fat disappear, but that didn't happen. After years of research and testing, they found that only a few people had a deficiency in leptin production. They also found that the leptin systems in most overweight people works exactly as it is supposed to work. The hormone levels climb when the person's weight goes up and falls when the person's weight goes down.

Somehow, this natural system of weight control has failed also. It seems that when some people reach the level of obesity, their bodies will not respond to supplemental leptin treatment. This appears to be especially true for people who have been overexposed to leptin. For some people, the leptin system works the way it should, for others it does not.

Also, researchers have found dozens of other hormones and peptides that are involved with appetite control. They are studying the new findings to see how the information can be used to help manage our eating habits and help us lose weight. In the meantime, we are getting bigger and bigger.

CHAPTER SIX

Nutritional Allowance for the Skip A Day Diet

GOOD WEIGHT LOSS plan should let you lose between two and four pounds per month depending on your activity level and diet. The Skip A Day Diet will allow that to happen, but you must follow the rules if you expect to be successful.

The Rules:

- You must consume between 1,600 and 1,800 calories on eat-day. Cut excess fats and eat lots of whole grain bread. This will give you a stomach full of nutrient-rich food at the end of the day.
- Do not eat excess sweets. You may have eggs, bread, lean chicken, fish (not fried), or sliced ham for lunch and dinner.
- No raw sugar (table sugar, jellies, jams, candy, or pastries) Exception: You may have jellies and jams on whole wheat or multi grain bread as part of the meal. Occasionally you may have a treat such as frozen yogurt with your meals.
- Between-meal snacks on eat-day can include multi grain bread with cheese, peanut butter, or other spreads such as pesto. You may also have a piece of fresh fruit.

- Eat regular lunch and dinner meals or have one large meal every other day. Most of your nutritional allowance should be consumed during dinner meals.

If you would like to lose weight rapidly, use this special nutritional plan. Eventually you will learn to skip breakfast and lunch as time goes by; in the meantime, use the menu shown below. The following foods are not likely to trigger your appetite and cause you to eat more than you should. Select your meals from the foods listed. You may also make changes to the list.

Eat-Day

Breakfast:

Cereal (dry or hot), Milk, Fruit, Pancakes (no syrup), Toast, and Rolls (coffee or tea)

Lunch:

Green Salads, Garden Salads, Asparagus, Chef Salad, Vegetable Dishes, Fruit, Legumes, Bread, Rolls, Crackers, Soups, Tuna Salads, Chicken Salads, Ham Salads, and Protein Dishes such as Veggie Patties, Tofu, Eggs, and Cheese.

Dinner:

Choose one from each group. You may choose another vegetable instead of legumes.
- Multi Grain Bread, Brown Rice, Pasta, Potatoes, Noodles
- Fish or Chicken (not fried), Turkey, Ham, Roast Beef, Steak, Pork Chop and Protein Dishes
- Green Beans, Green Peas, Spinach, Carrots, Cauliflower, Asparagus, Broccoli, Squash, Lettuce, Tomatoes, Mushrooms, Sprouts

- Lima Beans, Pinto Beans, Chick Peas, Black Eyed Peas, Black Beans
  Between-Meal-Snacks
- Multi Grain Bread, Cheese, Crackers, Cereal, Milk, Trail Mix, Fruit

Dieting Tips

- Drink one glass of water with each meal. Drink three glasses of water on Diet-Day, one at each mealtime.
- You can substitute a diet soda for a glass of water.
- You can substitute other related items not on the list.
- Sandwiches can be used for both lunch and dinner meals.
- Sauces, spreads, gravies, and salad dressings should be limited to the recommended serving size.
- You can mix and match the choices from lunch and dinner meals.
- You can have between-meal-snacks on eat-day.

Servings

Adjust the serving sizes to your appetite.
- One piece of fruit counts as one serving
- One slice of bread counts as one serving
- Vegetables: 1/2 cup is one serving
- Starches: 1/2 cup is one serving
- Meat and meat substitutes in ounces: 2 for lunch, 2 for dinner, 6 all day

The following is an example of the servings one might have on Eat-Day while using the Skip A Day Diet:

Breakfast	Lunch	Dinner	Snack
Milk	Green Salad	Bread	Cheese
Banana	Apple	Chicken	Crackers
Cereal	Bread	Potatoes	Milk
Toast	Soup	Vegetables	Fruit
		Pinto Beans	

The following is a breakdown of the number of servings one may have for one day.

Skip A Day Diet Servings in Groups

Groups	Servings/Day
Dairy - Milk, Milk, Cheese	3 servings
Meat/Protein - Chicken, Pinto Beans	2 servings
Vegetables - Mix Vegetables (2), Green Salad	3 servings
Fruit - Banana, Apple, Grapes	3 servings
Carbohydrates - Cereal, Toast, Bread, Bread, Potatoes, and Crackers	6 servings

Note: An allowance such as this would consist of about 2,400 calories over a two-day period. It would be about 1,200 calories per day for the two days. It provides about 90 grams of protein, which would give you about 45 grams of protein per day. This meets the recommended dietary allowance for protein.

CHAPTER SEVEN

The Skip A Day Diet, What to Expect

I T WILL TAKE a few weeks to get used to this new way of dieting. In that time you will balance your blood sugar and start bringing your metabolism back to its peak performance level.

During the first month you can expect to lose up to three pounds of body fat; during the second month you can expect to lose up to four pounds of fat. After the third month, you may continue to lose up to four pounds per month and your cholesterol and blood pressure will go down, provided you exercise.

Note: If you gain muscle from exercise, all of your fat loss will not show up on the scales as a weight loss.

Some months you may lose more or less depending on your diet and activity level. After ninety days, as your body becomes leaner, you will continue to tune-up your metabolism and lose weight. If you stick with your plan, you will be well on your way to reaching your target weight, and you will feel much better. You will be able to tell how well the program is working after about twelve weeks because you will have lost a noticeable amount of body fat.

During the first few days of the Skip A Day Diet, you will experience the symptoms that come with trying to quit bad habits such as smoking, drinking, or using addictive drugs. We call these symptoms withdrawal effects. Withdrawal effects are the body's attempt to let you know that it is time to eat or that you have missed a meal. While on the Skip A Day Diet, these effects may last only a short period of time and go away for good after a few weeks.

Some of the more common withdrawal effects are listed below:

Hunger
Crankiness
Get cold
Get light-headed
Have trouble falling asleep
Get hunger pangs in the stomach
Feel weak
Feel tired
Get backaches
Salivate when you see or smell food
Have headaches

The good news is that sipping water will, to some extent, eliminate withdrawal effects and satisfy the appetite. The symptoms may come on again at normal meal times, when you go around others who are eating or when you smell food cooking. Fortunately, withdrawal effects only require that you consume something, even if it is a liquid such as water and the symptoms will gradually go away.

If you feel weak, get dizzy, or have a headache while dieting, you might actually be sick. If the symptoms usually accompany missed meals, try the water first. In any case, if the problem persists, eat something to rule out hunger. If you don't feel better or the symptoms get worse, you probably should see a doctor.

If you have any health problems including diabetes or other illnesses, it is best to talk with your doctor before starting the Skip A Day Diet. Also, consult a doctor if you are pregnant, breast-feeding, or if you are taking medication.

CHAPTER EIGHT

Appetite Control

APPETITE AND HUNGER have basically the same meaning. Both describe a desire for food or something else. When it comes to appetite control, we may define both "appetite" and 'hunger" differently. We can say that there are three types of appetite and we can describe hunger as a real physical need for nourishment. The three types of appetite can be triggered by three different reasons: hunger, habit, and temptation. Hunger is a natural appetite trigger since it is a real physical need for food. When your body gets low on energy, your appetite will stay with you or keep coming back until you satisfy your hunger.

The habitual appetite comes on during times when you normally eat or when you are involved in activities that involve eating and socializing. The temptation appetite pops up when you are offered an unexpected, delicious treat that's usually free. Remember that ghrelin is present in your stomach at all times and may spike and trigger your appetite when your see food, taste food, hear someone describe food, or smell food cooking. Under the given definitions, appetite becomes more of a mental response. Since habitual and temptation appetites are psychological responses to food that may be brought on by something other than hunger, they can be controlled.

Things that may trigger the appetite include the following:

Free food	The smell of food cooking
The sight of cooked food	Rich desserts
Tempting snacks	Meal times
Break times	The sight of people eating
TV commercials	Pictures of food
Eating habits	Stress
Excitement	The inability to say "No thanks"
Treats	Social gatherings
Hunger	Thirst

Hunger might produce the strongest appetite response and trigger the appetite when you go without eating and deny your body vital nutrients or if you over exercise and reduce your glucose reserve. If the hunger appetite is suppressed too long, it could lead to binge eating. That is why your meals should include enough nutrients to satisfy your nutritional needs over a period of two days. Do not go more than forty-eight hours without eating a well, balanced meal.

Do not use fast food or sweets to satisfy your appetite. Use healthy snacks with bread and liquid until you can buy or prepare a healthy meal using fresh or frozen food.

Never use appetite-suppressing drugs as part of a weight loss program without a doctor's consent. So far, all attempts to put the task of weight loss in a pill have failed. Some advertisements claim that dietary supplements have the power you need to help you lose weight. Thus far, supplements have failed to be consistent. They are usually sold as natural products and are not regulated. This means that some supplements might help some people lose weight but not others. The correct dose for one person might be an overdose or under-dose for another person. To lose weight, you should use a diet/exercise plan, take dietary supplements such as vitamins, minerals, and phytonutrients to help restore energy and stay healthy.

Turning Off the Appetite

It would be much easier to turn off the appetite if we could fool our body into thinking we are full when we are not. That way, we could teach our brain to switch off our appetite at will. We cannot do that because the body has too many safe guards against it. However, there is a secret to turning off the appetite no matter how strong it gets. All you have to do is eat one large meal a day at random times of the day rather than having three meals a day all at specific times each day.

With this approach to eating, you will be able to decide when to eat rather than letting ghrelin decide your schedule for you. When you vary your eating times, you will be able to prevent ghrelin spikes in the stomach at certain times of the day. Remember that there is enough ghrelin in your stomach to spike and trigger your appetite at any time. By eating your main meal at random times during the day, you take control of your appetite. It's just that simple. One way to do it is to eat at between 3:00 and 4:00 in the afternoon on eat-day. Then you can have your snack on diet-day between 4:00 and 6:00 p.m. every other day. This way ghrelin will not have a pattern to follow at regular intervals.

After a large meal and a night's sleep, your body will recharge itself and restore its reserve using some of your stored fat. Actually, even if you do not eat a balanced meal before you go to bed, your body will still draw on your fat to replenish your reserve and turn off your appetite. The problem with not eating the day before is that the appetite will keep popping up throughout the day.

The next step in the process is to choose the food for your meals. Even if you eat only one meal a day, you can still gain weight if you eat the wrong type of food. In order to lose weight, you must fill your stomach with food that is relatively low in calories and high in volume. Your stomach should be full when you consume about 1,800 calories. Then there is the diet-day snack, which should be no more than 600 calories for the whole day.

This is a challenge because the stomach is about the size of a quart of milk. That's a lot of space for food that has been chewed and mixed with the fluids in the stomach. The stomach will relax and expand even further when digestion starts. During digestion, the stomach can expand to four times its size. People who eat for pleasure may continue to stuff themselves, long after their stomach gets full and digestion starts.

Since a full stomach can hold over 2,000 calories before digestion starts, never eat again after the stomach gets full the first time. Also, to ensure that you do not consume too many calories in nutrient rich food, you will have to reduce the amount of high glycemic/high fat foods and consume more bread. You may also consume low glycemic foods such as vegetables, legumes, lean meat, pasta, and brown rice. They will let your stomach fill up without going over your nutritional allowance. Also, they produce a constant flow of glucose into your system rather than flooding the body with sugar all at one time.

Don't be afraid to turn off your appetite because you can always take comfort in the fact that you are never more than a few cookies away from a hardy appetite.

CHAPTER NINE

Managing the Skip A Day Diet

THE SKIP A Day Diet, when done correctly, can be a safe and effective addition to your weight loss program. Diet-day is not fasting. Fasting is going for a period of time, usually a few days, without food and liquid. However, during a fast, a person will rapidly metabolize body fat if they consume water. Even while fasting and drinking water, a person can still lose only so much body fat. With the Skip A Day Diet, you can still drink as much water as you want each day and eat well, balanced meals every other day. This way you get the benefit of weight loss from fasting without really fasting.

If you need to lose a large amount of weight, take it slowly and be satisfied when you lose only two or three pounds per month. Eventually your weight loss rate will pick up as you become slimmer and more active. The slimmer you become the more fat your body will burn. The muscle you gain from exercise will help you lose weight because lean body mass is metabolically more active than fat.

As with any other diet, you may modify the Skip A Day Diet.

There are several ways the diet can be modified:

1. Eat light snacks (such as a green salad) before meal times on eat-day.
2. Eat your larger meal for lunch and a smaller meal for dinner.
3. Delay eating your first meal until after 12:30 p.m. on eat-day
4. Have some of your dinner meals without meat.
5. Have a healthy tomato-and-cheese sandwich for lunch.

There is no doubt that you, as a creative dieter, will come up with other modifications, so feel free to make adjustments to suit your needs.

In your pursuit for a healthy lifestyle, learn what you can from this program, follow the guidelines, and do the recommended exercises.

Managing Diet Day

Just like fasting, managing diet-day is both a physical and mental exercise that requires care and planning. Skipping a day of eating is much easier that fasting, but you will still have to deal with the problems people have while fasting. Over the years, they have come up with ways to manage the problems that come with missing meals. Some of the recommendations given for fasting, work well with the Skip A Day Diet:

1. Stay hydrated. Try drinking fluid throughout the day even if you aren't thirsty. Also, when you get the symptoms that come with hunger, sip water. Plain clear, cool water is best because it also helps control the appetite. If you prefer, add lemon juice to the water to give it a taste. Stay away from coffee and other drinks that have caffeine, because caffeinated drinks can be dehydrating and may trigger your appetite.
2. In all cases, try not to be sedentary during the day. Keep active, but do not exhaust yourself. If you normally work out in the morning, only do light stretching exercises and drink water

throughout the day. Strenuous exercise is not recommended on diet-day because you might become hungry and tired.

Managing Eat Day

The different foods you consume on eat-day could help your blood sugar remain stable and give you the energy you need all day on diet-day.

That is why it is important to eat a wide variety of food on eat days. While you are dieting, provide your body with enough nourishment to compensate for not eating one full day. Use plenty of whole grains breads, fruits, vegetables, and lean meat for protein.

Since it takes the body about twenty minutes to register when the stomach is full, stop eating when you have had enough. By eating more bread with your meals, you will put more stress on your stomach as it gives you volume. Do not overeat on eat-day in an attempt to make up for the food you missed on diet-day. Your body will have provided stored fat to help cover your nutritional needs.

You may want to experiment with different foods and eating schedules to find what works best for you. If you have trouble when you first start dieting, keep it simple until you find something that works. By eating well the day before, you will have enough nourishment to last all day on diet-day.

Give the Skip A Day time to work. Enjoy yourself and be patient especially when you have your meals with friends and family. Always participate and have fun but continue to manage your diet.

If you find yourself with extra time during the day, walk around and get fresh air, but avoid strenuous activity. You will actually feel better if you get up and move around occasionally rather than sitting at a computer or watching television all day.

Start eat-day by drinking fluids first, which will be absorbed quickly by an empty stomach. When you have dinner, start with soup and bread first. Then have the rest of your meal. Keep a record of the foods that work best for you and use them regularly. Pretty soon, you will have the Skip A Day Diet down pat.

The Skip A Day Diet makes sense for two main reasons:

You will have all the nutrients your body needs from day to day, and you will not be hungry. This makes the plan nutritionally sound and healthy. With successful weight loss, you will be pleased with the way you look and feel. When you have to face other health problems, you will not have to beat yourself up with guilt. You will not have to say things like, "I should have tried to eat healthier." This is how the Skip A Day Diet can help contribute to your success in having a good quality of life.

How to Break Old Habits

The best way to control your appetite while on the Skip A Day Diet is to remind yourself that it is not the day or time to eat. For instance, some people get up from watching television and automatically go to the refrigerator during commercial breaks. If you find yourself standing in front of the refrigerator with the door open, just say to yourself, **"Oh, I just ate yesterday."** This works most of the time. Other times you may grab a glass of water and take a few sips to satisfy your habitual appetite.

Stay away from places where food is cooking or where people are eating and do not take food that is offered for free. Consider this; a two-for-one special does not mean you should eat more. It means that the store can make more of a profit if it can sell two items and a soda at the same time to the same person. The sale is for the benefit of the store, not to help you. The price you pay will be for two items at a reduced rate. Nothing is free. You get what you pay for, and with fast food, you usually get more than you need.

Social activities and functions can be devastating to a diet plan because some people see it as a time to enjoy a free meal. While at social functions, learn to say "no" without offending the person who is pushing desserts and snacks. If you are at a party, and someone keeps insisting that you try desserts or treats, just say, "No thank you, I'm on a sugar-restricted diet." Most people will understand and will defend you if someone else tries to give you something you should not have. So, you will do much better in a group if you let others know about your efforts to lose weight.

CHAPTER TEN

Advantages of the Skip A Day Diet

1. The Skip A Day Diet will let you cut back on the amount of food you eat while keeping your diet balanced. This way you lose weight without depriving your body of the vital nutrients it needs each day.
2. It lets you include all of the foods you like in your nutritional allowance.
3. It gives the body time to cleanse and rejuvenate itself.
4. It gives you plenty of free time to do the other things you enjoy.
5. You lose twice the weight in half the time it takes with conventional diets.
6. You can have **occasional** treats such as pie, cake, chocolate, or frozen yogurt (if you must).
7. You can lose weight without strenuous exercise.
8. You don't have to starve yourself. Only eat when you need the food.

While on the Skip A Day Diet, you should be consuming more than 300 grams of carbohydrates on eat-day. This is more than enough for the average person because overweight people may need only 150 grams of carbohydrates a day or less.

CHAPTER ELEVEN

Managing Your Sugar

THE SUGAR IN candy is called sucrose, which is composed of two molecules: glucose and fructose. The molecules split and allow some of the glucose to enter the bloodstream as soon as it enters the mouth. This lets the brain receive glucose quickly when blood sugar is low. This action also causes the body to cut back on using stored body fat because sugar is an acceptable energy substitute for fat. If you continue to provide your body with sugar, it will have no need to burn stored fat.

If you are the type of person who does not eat very much but continues to gain weight, you could be creating the condition that causes weight gain. For instance, if you have an appetite for sweets, your body could be demanding the complex carbohydrates it needs to produce glucose. It may also be craving the vitamins and minerals that would come with complex carbohydrates. When you crave sugar, you might eat candy, cake, or other foods that contain sugar because your body has a need for glucose. Since the sucrose in these foods can act quickly to satisfy your appetite, you may not eat the complex carbohydrates you need to satisfy your body's demand. When you use sugar, sweetened foods to satisfy your appetite, it is only a temporary fix. After a while, your appetite will come back much stronger than it was before.

When you eat complex carbohydrates, always give your body enough time to process it and put it in storage where it will stay until it can be used as energy. To satisfy your appetite, eat a variety of foods rich in complex carbohydrates and eat a variety of vegetables such as broccoli, cauliflower, bell peppers, mushrooms, and carrots. You should include some of these in a salad for lunch and have some as part of your evening meal.

Remember to drink water with every meal and while you are exercising because it is the best drink for losing weight. Water dilutes and flushes the metabolic waste that is generated when fat is broken down and used for energy. By drinking water on diet-day, you will ensure that your metabolism remains high even while you are sleeping.

Sugar-Sensitive People

If you are super sensitive to sugar, you may find it more difficult to keep the pounds off than others who are not sensitive to sugar. Sugar-sensitive people, including those who have diabetes, have trouble storing the sugar from carbohydrates. If you are sensitive to sugar, get your complex carbohydrates from whole grain bread.

By eating one large meal a day, you will be better able to control your blood sugar level. When you eat only one large meal a day, your metabolism will slow down only once that day. Eating three meals a day will cause your metabolism to slow down three times a day. This routine can put you in a continuous loop of slow metabolism and makes it difficult to lose weight. Also, your meal can be spread out over two or three hours. This will ensure that your system will not be flooded with sugar all at once. After a large meal when your metabolism slows down, it will increase again only after most of your food has been digested. Digestion can take up to four hours.

Large meals that include simple carbohydrates will flood the body with sugar (glucose) every time you eat. Sugar-sensitive people cannot process and store glucose rapidly enough to remove it from the blood stream. They either need more time for the body to process and store the sugar, or they need to use insulin to help store it.

When your body is flooded with glucose, it is forced to continue to use sugar, never switching to fat, which is the preferred nutrient. This is the serious side of Syndrome X, which is also known as the Metabolic Syndrome. This condition interferes with the body's ability to process and store glucose. Syndrome X is more harmful to some people than it is to others.

If you are sensitive to sugar, you may have to use mostly complex carbohydrates for energy rather that simple sugars. By doing this, you will be cutting back on foods such a sugar, rice, potatoes, pasta, fruit and noodles and eating more whole wheat bread, legumes, and vegetables. This will help control the amount of carbohydrates you consume, thereby controlling your blood-sugar level.

Note: If you have diabetes, do not go on the Skip A Day Diet without permission from your doctor.

The Great Carbohydrate Debate

Scientists don't know exactly how many carbohydrates we need each day because we all have different energy needs. This leaves room for speculation and argument because people who are sensitive to sugar experience a metabolic slowdown even when they eat complex carbohydrates. Since there is no exact recommended dietary allowance for carbohydrates, it is a guessing game. The glucose from white rice can have an effect on sugar-sensitive people that is similar to that of table sugar, which is to raise their blood sugar level.

How many carbohydrates should we eat? When we look at the contents of a can of corn, we see that a one-half cup serving contains ten grams of carbohydrates, which is 4 percent of our daily carbohydrate allowance. This leads us to believe that we should eat 250 grams of carbohydrates each day based on a 2,000-calorie diet. Yet many researchers believe that the average person needs between 75 and 150 grams of carbohydrates per day.

It is possible that the estimation of 250 grams of carbohydrates a day is wrong. Since scientists seem to know that we normally need between 75 and 150 grams of carbohydrates each day, this gives us a starting point and a range with which to work. If a healthy, active 25-year-old man can manage with 150 grams of carbohydrates each day, a 25-year-old man who is inactive (sedentary) needs less. The person who is sedentary can manage with less because of his inactivity.

If 150 grams of carbohydrates per day is enough, then 250 grams might be way too much. Someone who is overweight, inactive, and whose body has a negative reaction to sugar needs much less carbohydrates. This lets us see carbohydrates from a different point of view. Instead of having carbohydrates supply 60 percent of our energy, maybe it should supply about 70 percent. This would mean the rest of the daily calories would consist of about 20 percent fat and 10 percent protein. If this is proven to be true, researchers may eventually change the carbohydrate allowance in the Recommended Dietary Allowance (RDA).

Nutrition and Carbohydrates

Carbohydrates are consumed and transformed into glucose, which can be used by the body as a source of fuel. This fuel is used for the brain, nervous system, and developing red blood cells. Glucose is also the primary fuel your muscles use when you start your exercise activities. At other times, the muscles use fat as their primary energy source for activity.

Your cells will readily use the glucose found in candy, soda, and cake, even though your body prefers foods rich in complex carbohydrates. This is important because processed sugar will upset your metabolic rate. Your body will constantly use stored fat and save glucose, especially while you are doing low intensity activities. Also, the body will continue to burn fat as long as you do not consume sugar. When sugar is ingested, the body stops using stored fat and starts using the sugar. The body is forced to use the sugar just to remove it from the bloodstream because it threatens to upset the blood/sugar balance. A constant blood/sugar imbalance could lead to more serious medical problems.

Glucose in the Body

While dieting, some people deprive themselves of carbohydrates and create a hunger condition. They eat small unbalanced meals that add up to less than 1,200 calories a day. The high calorie foods do not fill the person's stomach. In between meals the person gets hungry and may continue to snack on high-density foods such as candy, cake, cookies, or sodas. Active people who want to lose weight should eat larger, well-balanced meals before they get hungry. That is because food takes several hours to digest and become available for energy. Instead of using sugar sweetened foods for between meal snacks, use whole grain bread, vegetables, and other healthy snacks.

Raw sugar puts the metabolic system in a continuous negative cycle, a cycle that keeps your body from using stored fat. The amount of sugar that goes into the bloodstream is normally controlled when it leaves the liver. However, raw sugar and some of the sugar from starch can enter the bloodstream without going through the liver where it would be doled out in the correct amounts. This is why the body stops deploying and burning stored fat. Dieters can break this cycle by eating a variety of nutrient-rich foods including multi grain bread, vegetables, and lean meat such as chicken, fish, ham, and turkey.

CHAPTER TWELVE

Managing Your Fat

W HILE ON THE Skip A Day Diet, you will learn to choose foods that will keep your stomach full, and by managing your appetite, you could have a substantial weight loss in a few months. With the ability to manage and control your weight, you have to be careful not to abuse the diet and deny your body the nutrients it needs. As long as you skip a day of regular meals and have about 600 calories in snacks on diet-day, you will be fine as far as getting the proper amount of nutrients and fat your body needs.

However, when you start the full Skip A Day Diet and only consume water on diet-day, you might be tempted to cut too much fat from your diet. To prevent a fat deficiency, a minimum of 20 percent of the calories from your meals should be from fat. Since you will be skipping a day of eating, you should play it safe and keep the amount of fat from your meals at about 30 percent of your total calorie intake.

If you are consuming 2,000 calories on diet-day, about 600 calories of that meal should be from fat. Most of the fat you consume should be the so-called good fat, which comes from fish, poultry, and vegetables. Olive oil is also a source of good fat.

Do not make the mistake of thinking you need to cut all the fat from your diet because diets too low in fat may trigger cravings and cause you to go off the diet. Your body needs fat to back-up energy if your glucose reserve runs low. For instance, if you overwork on diet-day, your body will use the fat as a backup.

Fats also play other vital roles in the body. Fat is needed so your body can absorb and prevent deficiencies of the fat-soluble vitamins: A, D, E, and K. It provides flavor and texture to help food taste better and keeps them from being dry. It helps food stay in the stomach longer, giving a greater sense of fullness and preventing the return of the appetite. Fat may help your body produce endorphins, which are natural substances in the brain that produce pleasurable feelings.

On the other hand, extra fat calories in the diet convert to body fat immediately without much processing, where excess calories from carbohydrates and proteins go through a processing stage.

Also, several other things can happen if you cut too much fat from your diet. You may experience dry skin problems, hair loss, catch colds easily, have low resistance to infection, and lost of menstruation.

Gaining Weight

It's no secret that most Americans gain weight because of overeating and a sedentary lifestyle. A sedentary lifestyle is characterized by someone who has a desk job, watches television a lot, sits in front of a computer a lot, or spends too much time in social gatherings eating and drinking. The sedentary activities do not cause the weight gain by themselves. The person gains weight because of the amount of calories consumed and the lack of exercise.

When people are inactive, their bodies will not burn much fat, because only active muscles burn fat. Sitting causes weight gain because when people are sitting, their muscles relax and become inactive. When they stand up and walk around, their muscles become active again. So when they are in the sitting position, they take away the main metabolic process that continuously burns fat, which is muscle activity. A sedentary lifestyle makes it easy for people to gain weight, but the body has many built-in ways to keep them from losing weight.

The Body's Protective Measures

The protective measures the body uses to preserve fat are listed below:

- Low Metabolism
- Buffer Zone
- Binge Eating
- Plateau
- Constipation

The protective measures used to hold on to fat become stronger as you gain weight. This is why it is easier to get started losing an extra ten pounds than it is to get started losing an extra fifty pounds. Extra fat is just like a treasured gift to your body. It is not about to give up the fat without a fight. The first thing it does to hold on to its extra fat is to lower its metabolism. It wants to make sure that the extra fat stays on your body until you need it for emergencies.

Low Metabolism

Some people have a low metabolism and some people have a high metabolism. However, people who are at their ideal weight seem to have higher metabolism than those who are overweight. This means that as people gain weight, their metabolism slows down. By the time they gain sixty-five pounds of excess fat, their metabolism might have slowed down considerably.

If a man needs 2,400 calories a day to maintain his ideal weight, he would gain weight if he consumes more than the 2,400 calories a day. The extra weight will slow down his metabolism. After he gains weight, he would never be able to consume 2,400 calories a day and keep his same weight. His weight will continue to go up with the consumption of 2,400 calories a day.

As he continues to gain weight, his metabolism will continue to slow down. This will make his nutritional allowance obsolete for his age and height. His new nutritional allowance should be based on the amount of stored fat he has, rather than on his height because his metabolic rate would be lower. For instance, a man who has a certain height might have a nutritional allowance of 2,400 calories per day. However, because of his slow metabolism, he might need only 1,700 calories a day. If he continues to consume 2,400 calories a day, he will be getting 500 calories more than he needs. To keep from gaining weight, he will have to consume only 1,700 calories a day. To actually lose weight, he may have to cut his original nutritional allowance by as much as 50 percent. This means that he should be able to consume about 1,200 calories a day and let his body supply the other 500 calories from stored body fat.

This would give him a new weight loss nutritional allowance of 1,200 calories a day and would require a major lifestyle change. This explains why such a drastic change in the diet is necessary to lose weight. The old idea, of cutting back a few calories each day, does not work.

Your body operates as though its stored fat will be used to save your life someday. If you have tried dieting and failed, it is probably because of the efficient measures your body used to protect its precious fat. During a food shortage, your body will give out fat gradually because that is how Mother Nature has programmed it. Perhaps the fat will be used to take you through the coming winter when there will be little or no food available. The body will not give up its emergency reserve easily. Any food you consume during this apparent food shortage will be given the highest degree of protection.

As a woman gains weight, dieting usually becomes part of her lifestyle. She may start watching her weight as a teenager. When she starts dieting, her body puts up its defenses to preserve its excess body fat. When she starts cutting back on the amount of food she eats, her body reacts as though the time has come when there will be little or no food available; this is it! This is what it has been waiting for.

To protect its fat, the body lowers its metabolism even further in expectation of a long period of food deprivation. A determined dieter might continue to fight and lose a few more pounds at this point. This is no problem for the body because it has just begun to defend its stored fat.

The Buffer Zone

One of the protective measures your body uses against dieting is called the Buffer Zone. You have a Buffer Zone because your body keeps a 24-hour reserve of nourishment in its muscles and liver. If you are caught out in the wilderness overnight without food or water, the reserve will last until you can find food the next day, or about 24 hours. If you become trapped and you are inactive, the reserve will last much longer. Your body will start to use more of its stored fat and muscle as the reserve gets used up.

The reserve acts as a buffer when no food is available. When you eat again the body will replenish the reserve. Since your body can lower its metabolism, you might be able to starve yourself for up to seventy-two hours and not lose much body fat because of the buffer. However, you will lose weight.

The weight you lose while starving yourself will be water weight, because it takes lots of water to store the food you eat. Since you will not be eating much, your body will get rid of its water by using it to flush away waste. After the extra water leaves your body, you will see a dramatic weight loss. When you go back to eating regular, full-sized meals, you will probably gain more weight than you lost because your metabolism will still be slow and the water weight will come back. By the time your metabolism gets back to normal, you may have put on two or three pounds more than you lost while starving yourself.

After a diet fails, dieters may become more serious about losing weight. The next obvious step for them is to cut out all of the foods that make one fat. You might consume only light snacks because logic tells you the less food you eat, the more stored fat your body will burn. However, when dieters cut too much fat, carbohydrates, and protein from their meals, they are setting themselves up for a binge.

Binge Eating

You might experience a binge after you have been eating mostly foods like carrot sticks, grapes, and celery. The binge may be a psychological defense the brain uses to get you to eat. It seems that when people go on a binge, they have no control over their actions. Some dieters have been known to consume as many as 3,000 calories during an episode of binge eating. Apparently, the binge happens because the brain signals the body that food is clearly available; therefore the person should eat as much as possible while the food is there. The best countermeasure against the binge is to eat full-sized, balanced meals at least every other day.

The Plateau

When you finally get your diet working and lose a few pounds, you will probably be hit with another obstacle known as the plateau. The plateau can be a difficult and frustrating period of time because it seems that the body completely stops giving up excess fat during a plateau. It appears that nothing you do will let you continue to lose weight. Everything comes to a standstill, or so it seems.

At this point most people give up and go back to their old sedentary habits and ways of eating because they feel defeated. When they give up, they usually gain their weight back plus a few extra pounds. This is known as the ratchet effect of weight-gain. Your body holds on to its stored fat until you give up trying to lose weight, and then puts on the extra pounds, which will be used for the next perceived famine. This process is continuous; repeating time after time, diet after diet.

The plateau helps the body keep its fat and lets you continue to gain weight regardless of your efforts to lose. A plateau can last from four to twelve weeks, but it can be beaten. The key to beating a plateau is to consume food that is high in volume and low in calories such as whole grain bread along with very little meat, seafood, or dairy products. You will be rewarded for going through this hardship because after a plateau, you might experience a dramatic weight loss: a **real** weight loss.

Life does not get any easier as far as weight loss is concerned. As soon as you get over one plateau another one might hit within a few weeks. If you have a considerable amount of weight to lose, you might experience several plateaus before reaching your target weight. **Do not give up.** Deal with each plateau the same way. Be patient and continue to consume meals balanced for weight loss. Ultimately, the best way to handle a plateau is to continue to diet, exercise, hunker-down, and ride it out.

Constipation

When you start dieting, you might become constipated. This is expected by dieters and is accepted as a condition that comes with dieting. Doctors believe that constipation occurs because the person does not drink enough water or eat enough of the proper foods. To treat constipation, physicians recommend consuming multi grain bread, whole grain cereal, green vegetables, and other foods high in fiber. Dieters should also drink enough water to help prevent constipation.

You can see that constipation is not difficult to treat. It can be treated naturally with the proper high-fiber foods and liquids. Since this just happens to be the type of diet that dietitians recommend for weight loss, constipation can be just another way for your body to tell you to eat properly so you can lose weight.

However, if constipation persists or is accompanied by rectal bleeding, you should see a doctor because constipation could be a symptom of a more serious disease. It might accompany an illness that affects the tissues or nerves of the bowel, such as the growth of a tumor that partially blocks the intestines. It may also occur when a person uses laxatives too often.

Eat regularly to lose weight

To eat regularly is also an effective countermeasure against binge eating. Also, when you become overweight, your metabolism will have slowed down. When you start a diet, your metabolism will slow down even more. To prevent the second metabolic slowdown, eat at least one fully balanced meal every other day. When you start the Skip A Day Diet, you can have two meals on eat-day, a balanced meal for lunch and a balanced meal for dinner. Later, you will be able to skip the lunch meal altogether and increase the number of calories in the dinner meal. This keeps your body from experiencing a food shortage and slowing your metabolism. By eating regularly, your brain and body will know that plenty of food is always available.

The Skip A Day Diet

The Skip A Day Diet is the key component in this weight loss program. It lets you cut your calorie consumption in half and begin to lose weight. This is a direct countermeasure against the buffer zone defense system. By skipping a day of eating regular meals, you will be forcing your body to use part of its reserves. However, your body will not use all of its reserves, because this could lead to starvation if you actually had no food available. Instead of using all of your reserve, your body will use part of your reserve and part of your stored fat.

The Skip A Day Diet will act as a defense against the plateau because it lets you continue to eat well-balanced, full-sized meals, while keeping your total calorie count low. Since it requires you to skip breakfast and lunch and eat only one meal a day, the body will burn fat all day, until you eat your dinner meal. This will allow the body to use stored fat for energy while keeping your metabolism high. You may also use the Skip a Day Diet with Plain Food meals.

Plain Food Meals

Plain-Food Meals consist of common foods prepared without added fats, sauces, gravies, spreads, or sugars. The meals should be balanced with vegetables, high fiber bread, pasta, and legumes. Plain Food Meals may be supplemented with soups, and salads. Three examples of Plain Food Meals are listed below. The menu can be followed exactly as presented or used as a guideline when preparing your own unique meals.

Meal # 1

- One can of green peas - 3 1/2 servings, 210 calories
- Two slices of whole wheat bread - two servings, 200 calories
- One chicken breast without skin, baked or broiled – one serving, 284 calories
- One glass of water
  Total calories for the complete meal: **694**

Meal # 2

- One half can of green beans - 1 1/2 servings, 60 calories
- One half can of corn - 1 1/2 servings, 90 calories
- Two slices of rye bread - 2 servings, 200 calories
- Roasted turkey breast, 4 ounces dark meat - one serving, 211 calories
- One glass of water
Total calories for the complete meal: **561**

Meal # 3

- One half can of asparagus - 1 1/2 servings, 30 calories
- One can of spinach - 3 1/2 servings, 105 calories
- Lean, sliced ham, 4 ounces - one serving, 201 calories
- One cup of cooked, brown rice – one serving, 216 calories
- One glass of water

Total calories for the complete meal: **547**

You may use the following seasonings in Plain Food Meals: salt, pepper, seasoned salt, garlic salt, garlic pepper, and similar dry spices. Use mustard, ketchup, soy sauce, oyster sauce, and similar spices that have no fat or sugar. Do not eat Plain Food Meals all the time because they can be boring. Use them when you overindulge, hit a plateau, skip exercising, or the next meal after you have had dinner at a restaurant and gone over your allowance.

CHAPTER THIRTEEN

Multi-grain Bread, the Secret of the Diet's Success

THE SKIP A Day Diet lets dieters get away from the traditional dieting concept such as high fat, low fat, high carbohydrates, low carbohydrates, and lets the dieter focus on a staple food such as bread. When bread becomes the main course of the meal, everything changes. The dieter will be able to surround the bread with a variety of foods in the form of spreads and toppings. By using spreads and toppings, dieters will find it much easier to control the number of calories they consume from day to day. This gives them variety plus volume and brings into the diet a whole new range of food products.

With this approach to dieting, almost anything can become part of a person's nutritional plan. Everything from common cheeses to exotic foods such as caviar, anchovies, pesto, lox, and mint jelly can be part of the meal. This can make a meal much more enjoyable and exciting even when bread is the main course. It also makes preparing meals a much easier process.

All of the foods and spreads you choose will be used to enhance the favor of the breads you choose. This makes a lot of sense when you study it carefully. Multi grain breads have a low-glycemic food index, and you never have to worry about your blood sugar spiking above a certain level.

Once the diet is working for you, take it a step further and exclude processed foods that have chemical preservatives that may be harmful to you. You can also cut out processed sugars from your diet including table sugar, sodas, white rice, and white bread. If you want to tweak the diet even further, try counting calories. This will help you control the number of calories you consume. Check and see how many calories are found in your favorite loaves of bread. Then all you have to do is choose the low calorie spreads and toppings you like and use them on different days with different loaves of bread.

You can easily plan all of your meals in advance including the amount of protein and fat you intend to consume. You can include one piece of fruit and a handful of nuts with your meal every other day. A handful of nuts will insure that you get the good oils your body needs.

When you use multi grain bread as your main course, you will have the type of diet that most nutritionists recommend for losing weight. This diet is not complicated at all. Most people will be able to lose weight on a diet like this, which is exactly what we want to do, lose weight.

Always choose the denser loaves of whole-grain/multi grain bread because with the denser loaves, you consume more bread with spreads and toppings, which reduces your overall calorie consumption.

Whole grain breads, fruits, and vegetables make up a combination that is high in fiber, which pulls more water into the bowel. Good bowel health has a positive affect on your total body health including metabolism, cholesterol, and you will feel better altogether. Fiber also attaches to fats and other waste materials and removes it from the stomach and colon. It is the fiber in breads that removes excess fats and cholesterol from your body and helps to prevent constipation.

The trend now is to cut back on carbohydrates. Most people take that to mean stop eating all types of breads, but there is a big difference between breads produced with bleached flour and those produced with unbleached flour. Bleached flour produces white bread that doesn't have much fiber.

Scientific studies show that obesity is less prevalent in populations where the people follow a plant-based diet. Vegetarian populations worldwide, who use whole grain bread as the staple for their meals, experience lower rates of heart disease, diabetes, high blood pressure, and other diseases.

The bread stable is closer to our ancestors' diet than any other diet available today. This makes the Skip A Day Diet, with whole-grain bread, the ideal diet. All you have to do is add meat, vegetables, spreads, and toppings and you are on your way to a healthy lifestyle that you will be able to continue day after day, week after week, month after month, and year after year.

CHAPTER FOURTEEN

Exercise and the
Skip A Day Diet

WHILE ON THE Skip A Day Diet, exercise will help you lose more body fat and keep it off longer. As you slim down, higher metabolism will help burn excess fat. While dieting, do not over-exercise because it will cause exhaustion. Also, avoid fast-paced, high-intensity exercise because it will cause your body to burn sugar rather than stored fat, which can cause you to become hungry. The amount and type of exercise you do will determine the amount and type of energy you burn. To ensure that your body continues to burn fat, do low and moderate intensity exercises, and schedule your heavy workout sessions on your eat days. Otherwise, your appetite may return and force you to eat on the day you should be dieting.

CHAPTER FIFTEEN

Burning Fat with High Metabolism

Y OUR BASAL METABOLIC rate accounts for over two thirds of the energy you spend each day. The calories your body burns to support your basic life functions determine your basal metabolic rate. Those energy needs stay about the same from day to day.

This is the process that keeps the lungs working, the heart pumping blood, the muscles working, and the kidneys doing their job. All of these metabolic processes require energy. The energy transfer involved with processing and distributing food for nourishment accounts for about 70 percent of your metabolism. The other 30 percent is spent on work and exercise activities.

If you normally consume 2,100 calories per day in energy, 1,400 calories will be spent on metabolism, and the other 700 should go toward the energy you spend on daily activities. If you burn only 1,800 of the 2,100 calories you consume that day, the other 300 calories will be stored as fat. This is how you gain weight. To gain one pound, you must consume 3,500 calories more than your body can burn.

To lose one pound in seven days, you will have to burn 500 calories a day more than you consume (7 x 500 = 3,500). If you only need 2,100 calories a day to live, your body would have to burn a total of 2,600 calories each day (2,100 + 500) to lose one pound in seven days.

To get your body to burn enough body fat to lose weight, you must reach a certain level of fitness, which is a process that requires time, preparation, and training. Your body can burn an extra 500 calories in fat in one day only if it has been trained and conditioned to do so. The training should include physical, nutritional, and other measures that will get your body ready to burn the fat.

By using proper physical training and a balanced diet, you can burn a pound of excess body fat in seven days. All of the extra fat that you burn must come from exercise activity. Therefore, your diet must allow for maximum weight loss while providing the energy you need to function well above your normal activity level.

We now know enough about metabolism, exercise, and nourishment to make the assumption that you can safely burn an extra 500 calories a day by doing three, twenty-minute sessions or one hour of exercise. Most modern exercise machines will let you set the intensity and duration of an exercise session and record the number of calories you burn while exercising. To burn 500 calories during one hour, your intensity level should be about that of someone who is doing one of the following activities:

- Playing Golf (walking)
- Walking 4.5 miles per hour
- Bicycling 13 miles per hour

To condition your body to burn 500 calories in one day with activity, you must do both fast- and slow-paced exercises to build muscle density. The amount of muscle you gain will have an effect on your metabolic rate and your appearance. During the first part of your conditioning, you may gain weight from muscle build-up.

The amount of energy used for activity depends on how many muscles are involved and the intensity of the activity. The total amount of calories you burn will depend on the amount of work your muscles do during the exercise period.

As you gain muscle density, your metabolism will speed up. If you lose muscle density and gain fat, your metabolism will slow down. Metabolism will also slow down when you are not getting enough to eat or if you are inactive. If you reduce your daily nutritional allowance when you increase your exercise intensity, you may not have enough energy for all of your metabolic and exercise activities. It takes time to train your body to deploy and burn stored fat.

You cannot start and sustain a good diet and exercise program without proper nourishment. You can only have an effective weight loss program after you have conditioned and trained your body to use stored fat as part of your daily nutritional needs.

CHAPTER SIXTEEN

Fat Burning Conditions

YOUR ACTIVITY LEVEL, the food you eat, and the level of your metabolism determine the amount of fat your body burns. You must manage these conditions in order to make your body draw on its stored fat and use it for energy.

As long as you are including multi grain breads, vegetables, legumes, wheat, potatoes, and pasta in your meals, your liver will process the carbohydrates and store it as glycogen. The glycogen will be transformed to glucose and distributed to your muscles as needed. Since your liver can store only a certain amount of glycogen, your body prefers to use its stored fat for energy and preserve its glycogen.

As long as your exercise is not rapid and strenuous, your body will save its glycogen and use stored fat. Under these conditions, your body will continually take fat from storage and deposit it into your bloodstream where it can be burned as energy.

If you exercise twenty minutes or more per session and eat balanced meals, you will increase the rate at which your body burns fat. However, when you eat food with added sugar, excessive amounts of starch, or added fat, the fat burning conditions no longer exist. Everything comes to a screeching halt.

As soon as your body detects a certain level of sugar in your bloodstream, a message will go to the brain signaling that there is no longer a need to preserve your glucose reserve. Your body will stop using stored fat and start using the sugar. Also, when excess fat enters the blood stream, the body simply stores the excess fat into the fat cells immediately. It makes no difference if your body has stored fifteen pounds of fat or 300 pounds. The signals work the same for everyone every time. It makes no difference if the sugar you consume is table sugar (raw sugar), fruit sugar, or that from rice. The only sugar products that you can consume and have your body continue to burn stored fat is that produced from foods containing complex carbohydrates such as whole grain, and multi grain breads, vegetables, pasta, and brown rice.

When you use continuous exercise activity for burning stored fat, your intensity level should not be so high that your body is forced to use its reserve glycogen instead of its fat reserve. Yet, the intensity level should be high enough to burn enough calories so that you can reach your weight loss goal.

CHAPTER SEVENTEEN

Using Glucose and Fat to Fuel Exercise

WHEN YOU START an exercise session, your glucose requirements will increase. If your pace is too fast, you will over exercise and use up your glucose reserve quickly. When that happens, your muscles will consume all of your glucose, and you will become exhausted and feel hungry, tired, dizzy, or weak. You will begin to recover when enough glucose is provided for the brain, muscles, and nervous system. Over a period of time, your body will learn to store a larger glucose reserve for your daily activities including high intensity exercise.

If you keep the starting pace slow, your muscles will use some of your glucose reserves until your body can break down and deploy fat into the bloodstream. If you continue exercising at a slow, steady pace, after twenty minutes your body will have used up most of the glucose available in the bloodstream. When the exercise continues past twenty minutes, the body will shift to burning mostly fat for energy. This is the point where exercise causes your body to draw on your stored fat to satisfy its energy needs.

This is the perfect time for the body to use a lot of stored fat. From this point, your body will continue to draw on and use stored body fat for your energy needs. Even at rest, 60 percent of your energy needs comes from fat. As long as you do not consume more fat than your body needs for the activities you are engaged at the time, your body will draw fat from storage and use it. This is the point in the metabolic process where weight loss takes place.

However, as soon as you eat a meal that contains fat, the fat burning conditions stop. When incoming fat from your stomach reaches the bloodstream, it begins to replace the fat that is coming from stored body fat. When the level of fat coming in from the stomach reaches the level the body needs for its activity level, the body stops deploying stored fat. When the level of incoming fat in the bloodstream exceeds the amount the body needs for its activity level, the excess fat goes directly from the bloodstream into the fat cells. It's just that simple. This is where weight gain takes place.

Use Stored Fat for Distance

Glucose is important in anaerobic exercise, (high to extremely high activity), but stored fat is more important in aerobic exercise (slow to moderate activity). When you exercise at the higher intensity, you will be able to exercise for only a short period of time (eight seconds to three minutes) because the body can only produce so much glucose from stored glycogen during a certain period of time.

Your total glucose supply can be used up in about twenty minutes if the exercise is too intense. Untrained people will only be able to store a few minutes of glucose for exercise, but athletes will be able to store much more.

When you exercise at a slower pace, you will use more fat for fuel while exercising. Since your body will be using fat, you could go on exercising for many hours and not worry about running out of fuel.

When you are involved in an extended activity at slow to moderate intensity, your muscles will use more fat after a twenty-minute warm-up. Constant signals will be sent to the brain telling the body to continue to release stored fat. The muscles will use their stored glycogen to help burn the once stored fat. This way you can keep going on stored body fat, while using the glucose in your muscles to help metabolize the fat. This is why long distance runners can eat so much and not gain weight.

Since the body has the ability to produce some glycogen from protein (lactic acid and amino acids), you can survive with only a small glycogen reserve, which will help burn fat. The body can also change some fat into glucose, but you cannot starve yourself and expect to survive on stored body fat alone.

It is dangerous to try to burn only stored body fat because the body still needs outside nutrients. When trying to lose weight with exercise, keep a nutritional balance with enough carbohydrates for the energy you use. If you over exercise, your muscles will deny your brain the glucose it needs to function properly. This makes very high intensity exercise dangerous when you are not getting proper nourishment.

Stored fat can be broken down for use as energy by aerobic metabolism. The conditions under which aerobic metabolism take place are present during aerobic exercise, during long periods of food deprivation, and while doing light activity. You can (to some extent) create this condition by skipping breakfast and lunch and eating a larger meal for dinner.

By skipping breakfast and lunch, you will be signaling deprivation and encouraging your body to burn more stored fat. By eating a large meal once a day, you will have the nutrients your body needs to function properly the next day. The complex carbohydrates you eat will help metabolize and burn your stored fat on the days you skip eating. Remember that many millions of people survive on only one meal a day. The one meal may consist of only a piece of bread.

When you are resting, your body keeps a certain level of fat in your bloodstream. When you start exercising, the fat level falls because of usage. If the exercise continues for more than twenty minutes, the hormone epinephrine is released. This causes fat cells to begin rapidly breaking down their stored triglycerides and releasing fatty acids into the bloodstream. After about twenty minutes of exercise, the blood's fatty acid level goes up way past the normal resting level.

After the fatty acid level increases, the body uses fat as its main energy source. By doing slow, low intensity exercises first, then switching to moderate exercise activity, you can exercise continuously on stored body fat. Athletes can lose more than 10 percent of their weight in a 24-hour period under these conditions. Doctors and health care professionals will not allow professional athletes to lose more than 10 percent of their body weight because it is considered unsafe.

People who are not as physically fit as athletes should lose no more than 1 percent from their excess stored body fat during a 24-hour period. For example, if your ideal weight is 150 pounds and you weigh 200 pounds, you would have 50 pounds of excess stored body fat. One percent of 50 is 1/2 pound. You should lose no more than 1/2 pound per day.

For safety reasons, while using this weight loss program, never attempt to lose more than 1/2 pound in two days, whether you are trained or untrained. As your body and muscles become more conditioned, you will be able to lose more weight by keeping a consistent, steady approach to weight loss. By keeping a regular routine, you should be able to easily lose 50 pounds a year. Also, the body can be trained to use its stored fat more effectively as a fuel for moderate intensity exercises.

Since the intensity of the exercise you do affects the type of energy the body burns, try to go from low to moderate intensity exercises during a session. Since fat makes less of a contribution to the fuel the body uses for energy with very high intensity exercises, your exercise intensity level should be low to moderate. However, the level of intensity is different for each person. For a trained person, the intensity level could be moderate. The same level could be extremely high for an untrained person. Therefore, you will have to determine your own moderate intensity level.

Exercise to Get in Shape

The body needs more oxygen to metabolize fat for energy than it does to metabolize glucose for energy. Therefore, oxygen must be available for fat to act as fuel for exercise. When a person is physically fit, his or her conditioned heart and lungs will deliver enough oxygen to the muscles so the body can use its stored fat. To condition the heart and lungs, one should use aerobic exercise because it will help increase the amount of oxygen the lungs take in.

If you are breathing easily while exercising, your body will be getting the oxygen it needs for all areas. The easy breathing indicates that the muscles are getting enough oxygen to metabolize and use stored body fat for energy.

If you are breathing rapidly while exercising, your body will be required to use more glucose because you will not be getting enough oxygen for your muscles to burn mostly fat. This oxygen shortage will force the muscles to use glucose. The incoming oxygen will be used for other areas, such as the brain, heart, and nervous system, rather than for processing fat. You must keep your pace slow and burn fat.

How to Train Your Body to Burn Fat

The only way to train your muscles to burn excess fat is to use exercise. Untrained muscles use more glucose for energy, even when the exercise is moderate. Muscles that have been toned and conditioned through exercise are more dependent on fat and less dependent on glucose for energy. The exercise you do one day will cause the body to draw on stored fat and place it in the muscles for more of the same type of exercise the next day.

You can train your muscles to use fat by working out regularly and using a variety of exercises at different intensities. After a while your muscles will adapt to the changes in energy and learn to store more fatty acids each day. After you have trained your muscles and conditioned your body, you will be able to exercise for longer periods of time at moderate intensity levels that were once considered high. This will allow you to burn more body fat.

How to Avoid Exhaustion

If you continue an intense exercise activity long enough, the stored glycogen in your muscles and liver will become completely exhausted. When that happens, the liver will be able to produce only small amounts of glucose from lactic acid and certain amino acids. This action by the liver can provide enough glucose to keep you going. Other wise, you will be completely exhausted. You can prevent glycogen exhaustion by keeping a comfortable pace or resting before you become exhausted.

Without proper training and nourishment, the supply of stored glucose might be completely used up after one or two hours of strenuous activity. When this happens, the nervous system stops functioning properly. Distance runners use the term "hitting the wall" to describe this condition. To prevent complete glucose depletion, do the following:

- Eat meals rich in complex carbohydrates.
- Do not consume meals prepared with added fat.
- Condition the muscles to store more glycogen.
- Do not consume concentrated sweets such as candy, cake, or soda while training or after an event.
- Improve your cardiovascular fitness so your muscles receive the oxygen they need to burn fat.

CHAPTER EIGHTEEN

Aerobic Exercise

HEALTHCARE PROFESSIONALS ADVISE people who want to lose fat to do aerobics for a minimum of twenty minutes per day. You can accomplish this by jogging, walking fast, bicycling, swimming, dancing, or playing certain sports.

The longer you participate in the exercise activity, the more body fat your body will burn. If you can exercise for twenty minutes, three times within a few hours, your body will burn mostly fat during the entire time period. Then it will continue to process and use stored fat long after the exercise has stopped.

When you go to sleep at night, your body will draw on your stored fat and place it in your muscles to be used as fuel the next day. If you continue to increase the amount of exercise you do each day, your body will draw enough fat from storage so that you will be able to exercise more than you did the day before. If you increase the intensity a little each day, your body will make more fat available for your muscles each day. This process can cause you to lose weight. It is also the process that can cause you to gain weight if you do not skip a day of exercise. The body will lose weight on the day you skip exercise and gain weight on the day you have a good workout. Also, overweight people should skip a day of exercise just to prevent injury and exhaustion.

Slow to moderate intensity exercise is also better for overweight people because it is less stressful. Slower paced exercises with less stress will allow the person to exercise longer without injury.

People who exercise for extended periods of time as opposed to those who use fast paced and very high intensity exercises are less likely to injure themselves. This is important because even slight injuries can cause big problems in a weight loss program. Muscle soreness, pulls, and strains can cause you to slow down or quit an exercise program.

When your goal is to exercise for the purpose of burning calories, moderate intensity exercises will give better results than very high intensity exercises. It does not matter if you run for twenty-five minutes at a very high intensity or jog for fifty minutes at moderate intensity. You may still burn about the same amount of calories.

As stated earlier, the intensity of your exercise makes a big difference in whether you burn sugar or fat. If you exercise at a very high intensity for a short period of time, you will burn mostly sugar. If you go from slow to moderate, to high intensity exercise over a period of one hour, you will burn mostly fat. It makes a difference because the calories you burn in sugar will be replaced by your next meal. The calories you burn in fat **will not be replaced** as long as you eat balanced meals without added fat and continue to exercise. When you burn fat this way, it will be gone forever.

Your present fitness level will determine your exercise intensity level. While doing a sustained exercise activity, never run, walk, or exercise so fast that you have to stop and rest because of shortness of breath. When you have to stop exercising to catch your breath, you will be burning sugar. Your pace will be too fast. Just remember to pace yourself. However, you might be forced to stop exercising from the pain caused by lactic acid buildup before you get tired.

You can keep your pace at a level so that a few beads of sweat form and remain on your forehead. If you exercise inside a building that has air conditioning, you may not sweat at all. During a sustained exercise activity, your pace and intensity should be low enough so that you can carry on a conversation with a partner.

Keep in mind that you should exercise more than twenty minutes each session. Always try to plan your exercise periods for thirty minutes or more so that you will be sure to burn a considerable amount of fat.

CHAPTER NINETEEN

Neutralıze Your Sedentary Lifestyle!

A SEDENTARY LIFESTYLE is found mostly in modern, Western nations and is characterized by people sitting most of the day. As countries become more industrialized, the work gets easier, and the people become more involved in sedentary activities. This type of lifestyle and a lack of physical activity have led to overweight populations in many countries.

This pattern has resulted in many problems including the higher cost of medical care, health insurance, and many other problems related to obesity. As the obesity rate goes up in the United States, so does the cost of treating obesity related diseases and illnesses. This is a big problem because obesity related illnesses contribute to the rising healthcare cost and many deaths year after year.

Research shows that inactive people are more likely to die sooner than people who exercise and maintain a healthy body weight. Scientists who study the level of physical activity in people who died after the age of thirty-four have found that more than half of them die because of medical problems related to a lack of physical activity.

This makes a sedentary lifestyle as much of a danger to your health as drinking, smoking, or abusing other drugs. And it is all because of the obesity factor. Sooner or later, people who adopt a sedentary lifestyle usually develop obesity related diseases, whether their weight reaches the level of obesity or not. This means that being a couch potato can kill you even if you are skinny.

More and more plus-sized people are being diagnosed with chronic diseases like cancer, heart disease, diabetes, and respiratory ailments. Most of these illnesses are related to a lack of regular, physical exercise and are found in people who are overweight or obese. To get healthy and stay healthy, you must get into the habit of doing exercise and fitness related activities.

The average individual in the Untied States, who starts gaining weight after the age of twenty-five, will put on approximately one pound of additional weight each year as a result of inactivity. This does not seem like very much, but it will result in thirty-five pounds of excess body fat by the time the person reaches the age of sixty. These statistics are causing us to take a closer look at how and why people gain weight in the first place.

Not so long ago, the general consensus among healthcare professionals was that overweight and obese people gain weight because they are under a lot of stress, are compulsive eaters, depressed, or apathetic towards their health and wellbeing. Now, since almost everyone seems to be getting heavier, obesity has become a national problem. Both experts and the public believe something must be done to solve the problem. Some health care professionals believe that the effects of obesity are causing a medical crisis. This level of concern is causing the federal government to take a serious look at all of the problems related to obesity so they can come up with a solution.

Reducing obesity is becoming more of a national focus because of the growing expense. The United States government is feeling the weight of the financial burden that comes with caring for a nation of overweight people. More than one third of the adults in the United States are obese. Many others are overweight and will become obese.

The old idea of losing weight just by lowering caloric intake through dieting is not working. Scientists are studying our evolutionary past in search of solutions to our present problems. There is growing evidence that lack of exercise counters the effects of food deprivation. So a person can still gain weight while dieting if he or she does not exercise. Researchers are finding that diet alone (eating properly) is not enough to maintain a healthy body weight. We must exercise regularly: three times a week or every other day.

History tells us that our ancestors were highly active hunters and gatherers who spent the entire day searching for food in order to survive. Scientists recognize that we have been conditioned by millions of years of evolution, and during that time the human body became accustomed to a full day of physical activity. Our active past will not let us simply sit down and remain healthy. To keep our metabolism high and active enough to burn the calories we consume, we need a variety of exercise and lots of it. Also, without regular exercise we gain weight because the quality of our food keeps getting better.

For the first time in history, a majority of the adults in the United States are overweight or obese. This is a serious problem that's getting worse. Over 300,000 Americans die prematurely each year because of obesity related problems. If recent trends continue, it is only a matter of time before deaths from obesity related illnesses overtake the death rate from illnesses related to smoking, which total about 400,000 a year.

There is no doubt that physical activity is critical to the health of the human body. The body is tough enough to be used every day. The more you use your body, the stronger it gets. Each time your joints move, they move the muscles around them. This is how bones and tissue get their nourishment. With exercise, muscle density increases, flexibility returns, and the heart gets stronger even in older people. As long as you do not cause injury, the body will get healthier with exercise.

Your body parts are not like the parts in a washing machine. They do not wear out with use. However, inactivity causes stiffness in the joints, which causes atrophy in the surrounding muscles. This is one reason why bed rest can be deadly for people who already live a sedentary lifestyle. Bed rest does not make muscles stronger; it makes them weaker.

Heart failure is the leading cause of death for people over 65. At one time doctors thought that heart disease was a condition that came naturally with aging. Now they know that inactivity is putting people at risk for heart disease. This condition affects eight out of every 1,000 people over the age of seventy. The good news is that the condition can be reversed. Researches are finding that a good exercise program completely prevents or reverses stiffening of the heart muscles. This means that older people can have strong, flexible heart muscles and live longer just by exercising.

Another condition that affects older people who lead a sedentary lifestyle is arthritis. Researchers have found that a lack of vigorous physical activity in older people leads to this condition. This is a problem because a sedentary lifestyle is much more difficult to overcome when an older overweight person gets arthritis. Older, overweight people, who have arthritis, simply do not have enough strength and flexibility to exercise and lose weight. They generally get locked into a no-win situation. If they exercise, they are likely to injure themselves. If they do not exercise, they will continue to gain weight.

Nearly 60 percent of Americans who are sixty-five and older suffer from some form of joint problem making arthritis the leading cause of disability in the United States. Researchers believe that before long arthritis will afflict over forty million Americans. Eventually arthritis will jeopardize the quality of their independent living because of limited mobility. The condition of being overweight with arthritis will eventually keep the person from performing some of the basic tasks of daily living.

Arthritis causes problems with the following daily activities:

Preparing hot meals
Shopping for groceries
Taking medications
Walking to the mailbox

Getting in and out of an automobile
Dressing
Bathing
Using the toilet
Getting in and out of bed.

It is important for people to remain as active as possible so they can avoid a sedentary lifestyle. However it is easy to fall into a pattern of inactivity because of the pain, fatigue, and discomfort that come with exercise, especially for those who have chronic arthritis and other physical disabilities.

At the other end of the spectrum, juvenile obesity in the United States is rising rapidly. The incidence of obesity among children has more than doubled over the last 30 years. Now at least one out of every ten children between 6 to 17 years of age is overweight.

Children can get locked into a no-win situation as well as adults. Researchers are finding that juvenile obesity usually leads to adult obesity. Childhood obesity causes metabolic changes in the person who is overweight. These changes make the disease more difficult to treat when the child becomes an adult. Knowing this information might encourage children to make healthier food choices while they are still young. Children who learn about nutrition and apply what they learn usually have a drop in weight and have the knowledge and skills necessary to keep from becoming obese.

CHAPTER TWENTY

Sedentary Activities

THE DRIVING FORCE behind our sluggish lifestyle is the automobile, public transportation, entertainment, and other laborsaving inventions. These inventions that come with modernization are in the process of systematically eliminating exercise from our daily lives. This "lack of activity" is making us a sedentary society.

The two main activities that correlate closely with a sedentary lifestyle are television viewing and automobile travel. These activities have taken away our daily walking routines. Most people go from home to work by automobile. They work in an office building or factory that has a parking lot right outside the door. They use elevators and escalators instead of stairs.

To make matters worse, most people go to work at sedentary jobs, and 24 percent of Americans report that they do no exercise at all. After holding down sedentary jobs, which require them to sit behind a desk up to ten hours a day, they go home and spend countless hours watching television. This means they spend virtually no time engaged in physical activity.

It is not just the adults who are falling in to this trap. Children who watch television four or more hours a day are four times more likely to be overweight than those who watch less than two hours a day. In today's society, children are playing computer games, surfing the

Internet, and ordering pizza instead of playing basketball, running, or playing soccer. All of their sedentary activities are contributing to a huge surge in obesity.

A sedentary lifestyle can be a family affair especially when both parent work and the children are not involved in sports or other outdoor activities. Sedentary families usually spend a great deal of their quality time together in restaurants or other group eating activities. The food they choose usually adds to the problem because they buy the food they like rather than making healthy choices. This results in an inadequate diet, which is rich in sugar and fat.

In general, inactive children also consume large quantities of junk food. Consuming junk food and watching television for three or more hours of a day is one of the reasons there are so many overweight children in the United States. This is part of a typical sedentary lifestyle for both children and adults.

Parents purchase the latest computers, the best TV sets, video games, and whatever else their children need or want. All of these things contribute to and encourage a sedentary lifestyle. Parents who pamper their children only want the best for them, but they could be setting the child up for heart failure. Now, because of obesity, more young adults are getting heart disease and related problems.

Parents generally do not become concerned about a child's health and fitness until it is too late. Once the child has been conditioned and socialized into a sedentary lifestyle it becomes a habit. That is when it is the most difficult to get the situation turned around. Old habits are hard to break because by the time children develop a life of leisure, they are overweight and out of shape.

However, children can break their unhealthy habits and learn to make better food choices, but it takes time and education. Overweight children are generally not motivated to exercise, do housework, or go walking on their own. They simply do not want to give up the things they like to do. They become lazy and they like sitting around eating junk food all day long. That is the opinion of some researchers.

Junk food is an enemy for growing children. It is found within the home, in restaurants, and in schools. At home they eat processed foods, in restaurants they eat greasy, unbalanced meals, and in school they get their treats from snack bars and vending machines.

Junk food is also a convenient comfort food. When people become anxious, lonely, angry, or suffer from low self esteem, they console themselves with chocolate, soda, ice cream, cookies, and other delicious treats, which are usually high in fat, sugar, and processed carbohydrates.

It is not just the junk food. It's the main ingredients, sugar and fat, which keeps adding on the pounds. The average American diet now includes twenty teaspoons of added sugar a day. Much of this sugar is consumed in soft drinks, fruit juice, and other prepared foods. This, along with modernization, makes gaining weight easy. Caloric intake has gone up drastically over the past twenty years. In the United States, it has risen nearly 10 percent for men and 7 percent for women, while exercise activity continues to decline.

All of this makes it difficult to start doing the things we need to do to lose weight and stay healthy. It is not easy to just wake up one morning and start exercising and eating right. There are many imagined and real barriers that one must overcome before starting and continuing an effective diet/weight loss program.

Technology is one of the real barriers contributing to our sedentary lifestyle. We are not about to give up our automatic can openers, automatic garage door openers, remote controls, microwave ovens, elevators, or escalators. As more of these modern conveniences come into our lives, our active lifestyle deteriorates. Technology comes in and deletes the movement from our lives.

Besides these obvious challenges to overcoming a sedentary lifestyle, plus-sized people have other obstacles in their way. Exercise itself is an obstacle for overweight people because they have to deal with the pain, stiffness, fatigue, and the fear of injury that come with exercise. All of this also makes it difficult for them to gain the level of fitness that is necessary to burn excess body fat.

We can break our sedentary habits, but it will take education, time, patience, and effort. In the meantime our appetite for chips, cookies, chocolates, and other high calorie snacks continues to add hundreds of extra empty calories to our diet each day.

Another barrier to exercise may be the gym itself. A gymnasium can be a scary place for some people who are not comfortable participating in exercise activities with others. Crowded gyms can intimidate almost anyone especially overweight newcomers. This makes it difficult for a person to get started on a regular exercise program. Can you imagine walking into a room full of people for the first time? This can be a humiliating experience, especially when most of the people there are physically fit, and you are the most overweight one of all.

Injury is another barrier that one must overcome. Injury is not only detrimental to the individual; it can threaten the entire exercise program. People who injure themselves while exercising usually stop the program. However, older overweight people are the ones who are more likely to injure themselves while exercising because of the added stress. Naturally, if you injure yourself, you will not feel like exercising.

Over a period of time, a sedentary lifestyle will be harmful regardless of the person's diet. You can reverse the damage done by years of inactivity by starting and sticking with a good, regular exercise program. Even older people can start an exercise program and see amazing results within a few weeks. The common approach to weight loss is to simply go on a diet in an attempt to lose weight. Unfortunately, this approach does not work by itself. You will need an education in nutrition and exercise to be successful.

Sedentary Avoidance Activities

Activity can play an important role in helping people both lose weight and maintain a healthy lifestyle. Researchers are finding that exercise need not be strenuous for the person to have an active lifestyle. All you need to do is avoid sedentary activities. By avoiding sedentary activities, you become active. This means that you can lose weight just by doing housework, gardening, and fun activities such as window-shopping. Any type of activity can help with weight management.

People can avoid a sedentary lifestyle by finding other activities to take the place of the ones that require sitting. Following are a few ways to avoid inactivity without expending a lot of energy or doing vigorous exercise:

Sedentary avoidance activities:

- Park the car at the far end of the parking lot
- Do yard work such as raking leaves and mowing the lawn
- Do housework such as cleaning, vacuuming, dusting, and washing dishes
- Use stairs and walk whenever possible rather than using elevators, escalators, and moving walkways
- Walk during lunch breaks
- Use fewer laborsaving devices such as remote controls
- Play with your children or grandchildren
- Take a walk before breakfast or after lunch and dinner
- Walk or ride a bicycle to the corner store instead of driving
- When walking, pick up the pace a little each day
- When watching television, stand and stretch during commercials or ride a stationary bike
- When you want something, get up and get it yourself
- Walk around while talking on the telephone
- Stretch to reach items in high places and squat for items in low places

- Do not use the drive-through window at fast food restaurants (don't eat fast food)
- Do not take short cuts. Go the long way around when walking or shopping

Avoiding sedentary activity can be the critical first step for overweight people. From there they can move on to more serious exercises. This is especially true for those who cannot do a traditional exercise program. It is also a good start for those who simply do not like to exercise.

CHAPTER TWENTY-ONE

Sedentary Countermeasures

BESIDES THE DIET and exercise program, there are other steps you can take to help lose weight. Use the following countermeasures to increase activity:

- Avoid television or stand up and move around while watching
- Avoid long hours at the computer, get up and walk around
- Make brief appearances at social gatherings
- Take the stairs rather than the elevator all the time
- Walk to the store, post office, or library when possible
- Go dancing
- Learn Tai Chi
- Learn Pilates
- Go bowling
- Go swimming
- Practice Yoga

Countermeasures Summary

Both a diet and an exercise program are needed to counter a sedentary lifestyle and the body's defenses. The proper diet will keep you from gaining weight, and exercise will burn excess body fat. This type of weight loss program will force the body to draw on its stored fat, place the fat in the bloodstream, and burn it for energy.

With activity, the body will continue to burn fat as long as the person consumes food that promotes fat burning and avoids food that hinders fat burning. With the proper food, the body will burn fat when the person is involved in light activity such as walking or housework. However, even with the body burning fat continuously, you may not lose much weight.

Since the body has such a fantastic system in place to protect body fat and prevent weight loss, how does one lose weight? How can you win?

You can win by learning how the body handles and processes food, how it protects body fat, and by using countermeasures to overcome your system's protective measures. The following countermeasures can be used against those protective measures:

- Eat vegetables, multi grain bread, legumes, and fruit. They keep your metabolism high.
- The Skip A Day Diet helps overcome the body's buffer zone defense system and a plateau.
- Do not over exercise and trigger your appetite.
- Exercise to speed up metabolism.
- Balanced meals can be used to help control the appetite.
- Plain Food meals can cut calorie consumption.
- Use high fiber meals to help prevent constipation.
- Use activities such as housework, car care, yard work, and play to counter a sedentary lifestyle.

All of these activities work as countermeasures against different protective measures. Use all of the counter-measures as much as possible because no one countermeasure can be used exclusively against a particular protective measure.

If you are working full-time, raising a family, or running a business, it might be difficult to find time for exercise. However, the Skip A Day Diet makes the time available to you. You can start by walking during meal times on diet days. If you have a sedentary job, plan to do most of your exercises before or after work.

When you skip a day of eating, you set precedence for your body. You will be empowered by the Skip A Day Diet because you will realize that you do not have to eat every time you have a **slight** appetite. You will learn that if you can skip eating a whole day, you can learn to cut back on foods high in sugar and fat. This brings a whole new dimension to dieting. It gives you the power and knowledge you need to take control and manage your weight.

Losing weight is a battle you must fight with yourself. However, you **can** win the battle, but it **will not be easy,** and you **will** need help. That's why you are invited to visit www.skipaday.com to find other weight loss resources.

CHAPTER TWENTY-TWO

Exercise and Metabolism

ASIDE FROM THE energy needed to keep you alive and healthy, there are three types of energy expenditures that help determine your metabolic rate:

1. Energy spent while resting.
2. Energy spent in digesting food.
3. Energy spent while doing physical activities.

By following a few simple instructions, you can learn to use all of these metabolic activities to your advantage for maximum weight loss. Your resting metabolic rate will go up; the energy you spend while exercising will increase, and the food you eat may cause you to burn more calories.

A person who is physically fit burns a lot of fat all day long not just during an exercise session. A one-hour workout in the morning could cause your body to burn fat all day because your metabolism will remain high — as much as 25 percent above average for up to three hours after a good workout. The body will continue to burn fat the next day because of that one-hour period of exercise. This is called the continuous exercise effect. Your body will still be actively burning fat long after you stop exercising. Never eat candy, cookies, or ice cream after an exercise session. Also avoid sugar-sweetened drinks and foods that contain lots of fat. If you do, you may lose the continuous exercise effect.

Using Physical Activity for Appetite Control

Exercise can delay hunger. After a good exercise session, it is not necessary to rush to the nearest restaurant and fill up on your favorite food because you will not be hungry. While you are exercising, your body will take nutrients from storage and flood the bloodstream with glucose and fat. These nutrients will help suppress your appetite while you are active. After an exercise session, you will have time to cool down, relax and rest before you get hungry again.

During an exercise session, the body floods the bloodstream with glucose and fat so that energy will be available for the exercise. After a good workout, the body continues to burn fat just as if you were still exercising. Also, while you are exercising, the body will stop digesting any food you may have eaten before starting the exercise session. Your body will start back digesting food again when you stop exercising.

When you relax and rest after a long exercise period, your body will take the excess glucose and fat from the bloodstream and place it back into the muscles and liver.

Note: Intense exercise causes huge energy expenditure and may stimulate the appetite to make up for calories burned while exercising. Therefore, you may have a strong appetite if you over exercise and reduce your glucose reserves.

Lose Weight by Increasing Activities

When you gained weight, it probably came on slowly. You might have gained all of your excess weight at between two and five pounds per year. The causes of weight gain vary widely among people. Some of the reasons are listed below:

- Environmental (family and friends who love to eat)
- Behavioral (inactivity)
- Psychological (eat when you get upset or depressed)
- Biological (medical problems)
- Genetic (inherited fat genes)
- Metabolic (thyroid problems)
- Dietary (unbalanced diet, no veggies, whole grain, and excessive sweets)

People can gain weight because of fast food, too much television, thyroid problems, inherited fat genes, or a combination of the reasons listed. Many children gain weight because of overindulgent parents, where treats and fast food are concerned.

If your weight gain resulted from any of the reasons listed above, you can lose weight by avoiding raw sugar and excess fat and raising your activity level. This will allow you to reverse the weight gain process. By eating a balanced diet and exercising in twenty-minute sets every other day, you should be able to lose twenty to fifty pounds per year.

Lose Weight with Exercise

When you start an exercise program, you will start building muscle density as soon as your activity level increases. As your muscle density increases, they will demand more energy. Because of the increase energy usage and muscle density, you may go through a period of time before you see results from your hard work. Depending on your level of fitness, you may go as long as twelve weeks before you see a real weight loss from your program. In the meantime, you will lose body fat and experience a weight shift.

In the beginning you will be starting slowly while doing only light exercises at low to moderate intensity. This may result in very little weight loss from exercise. You might even have a slight weight gain because it is possible to gain muscle density faster than you lose body fat. Since lean muscle is much heavier than fat, your scales might show a weight gain. This will probably be a shift in your body weight.

The weight shift will occur because you might be consuming a full nutritional allowance, which will allow you to gain the muscle density you need. Since you will be gaining muscle from the exercise, your body will be storing extra nutrients to support the growing muscles. The increased muscle density will allow you to continue to exercise every other day at a slightly higher intensity level. It is this dynamic process that may cause a noticeable weight gain in the first few weeks.

The temporary weight gain is enough to cause some people to quit the program. If nothing else, it might raise their frustration level and cause them to exercise more. Since they will not be losing weight, they might think that they are not working hard enough and will be tempted to put more effort into exercise. Strong determination such as this may result in more of weight gain and cause exercise burnout. When you feel that the weight loss program is more trouble than it is worth, you might just give up, especially if you have nothing to show for your work.

The weight you gain while on this program might be similar to the plateau dieters experience when they first start a diet/exercise program. They start with a reduced nutritional allowance and experience a temporary weight loss right away. After they lose a few pounds, their activity level increases, which encourages them to become more active. As they become more active, they gain muscle mass, which causes a weight shift rather than a weight loss. They refer to this point in a diet as their six-week plateau.

Dieters usually give up before they get over the plateau. This happens most often to people who do not understand the dynamics of weight loss and exercise. They are likely to say, "Hey, I am dieting and exercising but still not losing weight. What's happening?"

After you have been on this weight loss program for a while you may see the results in the mirror long before you see it on the scales.

You will look and feel better and see other positive changes about yourself. You will be more comfortable in your surroundings, and your clothes will fit better.

When you first start a weight loss program, the only way you will be able to tell that you are actually losing body fat is by your "Body Mass Index" (BMI). Your body mass index is how you look compared to how you should look according to your ideal weight. If you look like you have lost weight, but haven't, you probably lost stored fat and gained muscle mass. If you look like you have gained weight, you probably have gained body fat.

Keep in mind that weight reduction is a long, slow process. Be realistic in your expectations and think logically about what is happening to your body. If it took one year to gain five pounds, it is not likely that you will lose five pounds in two weeks. When you rev up your metabolism and exercise enough to burn an extra 3,500 calories over a period of time, you will lose one pound of stored body fat. The exercise for this task can be spread out so that you lose one or two pounds per week or one or two pounds per month. However, people who are physically fit can exercise enough to lose two pounds in a week.

If you continue to diet and exercise, your body composition will change from a fat form to a more lean form. Make sure you use a sensible exercise plan that will help you burn the maximum amount of fat for the time you spend exercising. Never do exercises that are too stressful because they might cause injury, and never over exercise because it might lead to burnout. Do not do heavy exercise sessions on diet-day because it might trigger your appetite and cause you to overeat.

According to all fitness experts and researchers, your body goes into a fat burning mode only **after** you have been exercising for twenty minutes. In the areas of fitness, exercise, weight loss, and conditioning, experts find many things on which to disagree: What to eat, how much to eat, and what exercise program is better for you? However, none of them disagree on how long it takes before the body starts burning fat after you start exercising. It is not nineteen or twenty-one minutes. They all agree that it takes twenty minutes. There is probably some latitude, but given this strong point of agreement among researchers, you should make your exercise sessions a minimum of twenty minutes.

You Can Burn More Calories Walking at 2 MPH, Confirmed!

Researchers at the University of Colorado at Boulder confirmed that people burn more calories per mile walking at two-miles-per-hour than walking at a moderate to brisk pace of three- to four-miles-per-hour. Researcher Ray Browning said that walking slowly burns more calories per mile due to moving more weight over the same distance as that of a skinny person.

See Reference Note in back of book: A paper by Browning

Compare Fast and Slow-Paced Exercises

Compare the differences between the amount and type of energy used while walking and running by overweight people and non-overweight people.

Normal Weight Example:

A 150-pound man who runs one mile in six minutes can burn 103 calories in mostly sugar.

A 150-pound man who walks one mile in fifteen minutes can burn 103 calories in mostly fat.

Overweight Example:

A 220-pound man who runs one mile in six minutes can burn 150 calories in mostly sugar.

A 220-pound man who walks one mile in fifteen minutes can burn 150 calories in mostly fat.

How Fat Reduction Works

Active people who have high metabolism can process and use more than seventy grams of fat per day. (Seventy grams of fat is equal to 1/4 cup of oil).

An ideal nutritional plan would allow your body to use the 70 grams of fat from your stored body fat, so that you will not have to eat fat in your meals, but some outside fat is necessary. High metabolism and exercise will allow your body to burn even more stored fat. In 30 days you could burn up to 4 pounds in excess fat just from high metabolism and light exercise activity. In six months you could lose about 24 pounds of fat. This is a safe and healthy weight loss goal and the weight will stay off. Therefore, it is safe to suggest that you can take in 35 grams of fat per day and still lose up to three or four pounds per month if you are active.

Since the body needs carbohydrates to burn stored fat, you will have to include enough carbohydrates in your diet to burn the fat released into your bloodstream.

CHAPTER TWENTY-THREE

Neutralization Activities and Exercises

P ART OF AMERICA'S inactivity problems stem from the progress we have made in improving our way of life. Over the years we have become successful at growing and preserving food, developing modern means of transportation and eliminating much of the strenuous work from our jobs. These modern conveniences have made life easier for us and have resulted in a lifestyle that we are not willing to give up. It makes no difference how fat we become, how much of the population has diabetes, or how prevalent heart disease is — we will not give up our sedentary way of life easily. We will continue to overindulge in delicious meals, opulent desserts, and scrumptious treats.

We have our favorite inactive or diet sabotaging activities: movies, television, Internet, social functions, restaurants, and we use much drive time to get to all of our mandatory functions. This is how our needs and wants create obstacles to our exercise activities.

- We have to see the latest movie, and we have to get the popcorn-candy-soda combo, which saves us money.

- We have to watch our entire football game, basketball game, tennis match, golf game, or baseball game. We have to have sodas, chips, nuts, and dip while watching television (none of that diet stuff).
- We cannot go to a restaurant and just have the meal. We must have a couple of drinks. We have to have appetizers. We must have dessert (Chocolate to die for!).
- We must have the two-for-one special at fast food restaurants. We must have the super-sized soda. We have to have the super-sized fries. We have to have the super-sized apple pie. We must have the double cheeseburger (and we must have it our way).
- Where has all of the time gone? We still need to check our e-mail. Since we are on-line, we have to read the news. We have to read the financial report. We have to see what is playing at the movies. We have to see the movie trailers. We have to catch up on sports. (Hmmm! Something free? Let's click here!)

This is who we are and the things we do. How can we overcome this problem?

This leaves only one solution, and that is to find a way to neutralize the effects of our sedentary lifestyle without actually giving up the things we love to do. With all of the sports and movies to watch, with the need to eat three full-sized meals a day, and with the need to search the Internet, we simply do not have time to exercise. With so many demands, where do we find time for physical fitness? You can start exercising with all of the free time you get from going on the Skip A Day Diet.

CHAPTER TWENTY-FOUR

Beat Obesity Boot Camp

BEAT OBESITY BOOT Camp is composed of a series of workshops designed to educate both parents and children about childhood obesity and the problems and illnesses associated this disease. The activities and discussions associated with the boot camp will give the parents and children a chance to talk about dieting, exercise, overeating, and childhood health. Workshop discussions will give them an opportunity to learn how overweight children feel about being overweight. It will also let them know that they are not helpless when it comes to managing their weight and health.

Children will learn that there is a big responsibility involved with taking care of themselves. The workshops are designed to give older children and young adults an opportunity to take over the responsibility of their own health and weight management. They will learn that the things they do while they are still young will effect how they look and feel when they get older. The things they do now may even determine how long they live.

When children become armed with this knowledge, it will be up to them to start making the right choices for themselves.

The boot camp is a resource for parents and kids. It consists of several topics for discussion that you may find online at skipaday. com. You may copy, rewrite, and modify the workshop material for your particular needs. Also, you may build on Obesity Boot Camp in designing your own boot camp for kids.

Intervention Workshop for Children

To conduct workshops, choose a facilitator who can guide the discussion and keep the group on track. Small group workshops of about ten to twelve people will give everyone a chance speak and respond to comments. The groups can be mixed with both parents and children or they can be just parent or just children with an adult facilitator. The goals of the discussion should be to give the children an up-close and personal look at themselves, from the point of view of other children and adults. This will let everyone there know that overweight children are just like everyone else. They care about being overweight, and they are sensitive about how they look. They notice when people are staring, teasing, or talking behind their backs. Also, the group will learn that being overweight is not the child's fault. It is generally the parents' fault. When a facilitator brings the facts out in a discussion, parents might admit that they should do a better job of managing their children's diet and health.

The facilitator may guide the discussion by asking questions and keeping the group focused. Otherwise, things will get off track. The facilitator can use questions that give both parents and children an opportunity to talk and express their feelings on different subjects.

Facilitator Managed Group Discussion

Sample Discussion Starters:

Facilitator speaking to the group:

* We are having this discussion regarding children who are overweight because we want to find solutions to the problems

and you can help. We want to show that people, who are overweight, are just like everyone else. I want to get the point across that overweight kids are regular boys and girls.

* I will be asking questions of each of you and giving you a chance to add to the discussion with your comments. That way we will get to know how you feel about the issue of obesity in children and what we can do about it.

* Before we get started, let's get to know each other. We will go around the table (room) and give each of you a chance to introduce yourselves and tell us what you enjoy doing for fun.

* Optional: Tell us what you like about school and what you would like to do when you grow up: doctor, lawyer, dentist, teacher, fireman, actor, or police officer.

* Since this discussion is about overweight children, I will ask you some questions directly in regards to being overweight. Also, if you are not overweight, I will ask you similar questions regarding overweight children you may know. I will also ask parents questions related to their own children or other children they know.

Questions for Children

1. How does being overweight bother you?
2. Is being overweight a problem for you?
3. Is your weight a problem for other people with whom you come into contact?
4. Do you think there is a problem with being overweight?
5. How do you think you got to be overweight in the first place?
6. What are your favorite foods?
7. What are your least favorite foods?
8. If you could lose all of your excess weight and get down to your correct size, what would you do to keep the weight off?
9. If you could give a message to other young children to help keep them from getting overweight, what would you tell them?

Questions for Parents

1. Is it easy to say no to your children when it comes to giving them what they want?

2. Do you have a clear enough understanding about nutrition to make the best food choices for yourself and your children?

3. Would you be willing to learn what it takes and try it with your children if it means better health for them?

4. If you could start over in managing your children's weight, what would you do differently?

5. When given a choice, what type of food do your children choose that is healthy or unhealthy?

6. Do you think children would refuse to eat and holdout until they get what they want?

7. Do you think that if you sat down and had a long talk with your children about making the right food choices that they would understand and cooperate?

CHAPTER TWENTY-FIVE

Childhood Obesity, Intervention Workshop

When it comes to obesity, Education is the Key to Prevention
The solution is good childhood healthcare.

Group Lecture

I NTRODUCTION: IF YOU'VE been reading the newspapers or listening to the news, you know that childhood obesity is getting to be a major problem in the United States. Over one-third of our population is overweight. This is alarming because younger people are getting diseases and illnesses that are directly related to obesity. They include heart disease, cancer, stroke, and kidney disease. As the rate of obesity goes up, so does the cost of health care. If the trend continues, over the next ten years, one-third of the children growing up today could be suffering from obesity and have a shorter life-span than their parents.

Normally when we see news reports of overweight children, the pictures show only the overweight bodies but not their faces. But there is much more to overweight children than the fat they carry. They are real people with hearts and souls. They are sensitive about their weight and they get their feelings hurt more often then other children.

Throughout this program, you will meet some of those overweight children and get to know them. They may even tell you how they feel about being overweight. Try to understand that this is not an individual problem; it is a national problem.

We can't afford to wait around until our children get old enough to learn to manage their health on their own. They need to start developing good health habits now. They also need to know that exercise and a healthy lifestyle can extend their lifespan. Also, we have to teach parents and make them understand that what they do now will have a tremendous impact on their children's lives.

Since the cycle of obesity revolves around poor eating habits and incorrect food choices, we can stop the cycle by developing good eating habits and making better food choices for our children. If we don't stop it now, we will in fact be killing our kids by letting them continue the cycle. It will not be easy, but we can do it.

Culture can play a big part in weight-gain. Most of our social and cultural activities involve eating and drinking. Some might take not eating while attending a social function as antisocial. Children might feel that mom; dad, aunty, or uncle may become upset if they don't eat very much. That is one reason why some children overeat. They want to please others while participating in social activities.

Overweight parents who have overweight children may make the wrong choices for themselves and their children. In some cases, parents simply leave it up to the children when it comes to food choices. In cases such as that, a child may make the wrong choice or overeat because no one has taught him or her what to eat or that it is unhealthy to eat too much.

Children usually grow up following the eating habits their parents allowed them to establish for themselves. Or the children simply eat and enjoy the same types of foods their parents enjoyed. Unfortunately, too many of the parents today grew up with fast food as their number one choice. Their children are following in their footsteps.

Children are dependent on their parents to make correct decisions for them. A baby does not know that eating excess calories could lead to health problems and an early death. If you allow your child to have excessive amounts of candy, ice cream, and fast food, they have no way of knowing that when they consume sugar in excess, it's bad for their health. Children eat whatever their parents give them or allow them to have.

Most parents provide for their children's needs including a good home environment and entertainment such as video games, television sets, computers, and lots of toys. Some parents will let their children have whatever they want, whether it's healthy or not. When given a choice, a child will choose sweets and fast foods over healthy food every time. Managing your children's weight and teaching them to eat for good health is a difficult job. It takes tough love to keep your children healthy.

It is not easy to make your child eat whole-wheat bread, vegetables, legumes, and drink water with their meals when everyone else is having hamburgers, fried chicken, pie, ice cream, cookies, and sodas. Your children will refuse baked chicken, baked fish, homemade vegetable soup, whole wheat bread, and brown rice. They will even turn down a ham sandwich with lettuce and tomato for something better.

The logic is simple. If certain foods taste better, why eat something else. When given a choice, a child will choose hamburgers, French fries, cakes, cookies, ice cream, doughnuts, sodas, juice, and candy. Food choices should not be up to the children. It should be up to their parents until the children learn to be responsible.

If parents let children make the choices, the children are likely to gain weight and get illnesses and diseases related to obesity. This will shorten their life span. There is no question about it. People, who are overweight, generally die sooner than those who maintain a healthy weight and a good level of fitness.

You might be able to add five to ten years to your children's life just by teaching them to eat healthy food rather than letting them make bad food choices. Yes, you have to make the choices, especially if the children have made bad choices in the past. Will it be easy?

No, but tough choices are what it is going to take to manage your children's health.

If they are use to making food choices for themselves, they will do everything they can to make you give them what they want:

They will scream
Throw temper tantrums
Jump up and down
Throw food away
Turn their plate upside down
Curse and swear at you
Refuse to eat anything at all or
Accuse you of being mean, uncaring, and abusive

Will this bother you? Sure it will! If your child acts up enough, chances are, you will give in. It is human nature to be a good parent. Also, you don't want to be accused of abusing your children.

However, if you let your children win the argument; they are the losers in the long run. When they become obese as a minor, the stage is set. They are not likely to recover from obesity as an adult. Regardless of the excuses one might have for allowing their children to become obese, it is ultimately the parents' responsibility. When you give in and let your child make bad food choices, you are killing your kid with kindness.

CHAPTER TWENTY-SIX

Large Group Workshop for Parents

To conduct a large group workshop, ask members of the community to help out as facilitators and presenters. Use the following guidelines to build and arrange the workshop the way you want: Choose the subjects that you want covered during the workshop and provide the facilitators and presenters with guidelines and instructions. The presenters can do the research and put their own presentation together within the allowed time period. Include teenagers as presenters when possible.

Presenters may be nutritionists, doctors, personal trainers, community leaders, fitness experts, concerned parents, or people who have lost weight. Different presenters may cover different subjects.

Subjects for Discussion:

* Childhood obesity, a cause for alarm
* Food facts, too many bad choices
* Statistics, Obesity across America
* Trends, Where are we headed?

Presenter 1: To cover childhood obesity

* What is childhood obesity? Why should we be concerned? What causes obesity in children?

Presenter 2: To cover food facts and too many bad choices

* The average child needs how many healthy calories each day? The average child consumes how many unhealthy calories? What are healthy food choices? What are unhealthy food choices?

Presenter 3: To cover statistics, obesity across America and your state

* When did childhood obesity get to be a problem? What was it like ten years ago? What is it like now? What about obesity in adults?

Presenter 4: Trends: Where are we headed?

* What can we expect unless something is done to stop the problem? What is the outlook on our national health? How will obesity affect our healthcare system in the future?

Workshop #1, Topics for Discussion

Narrator's research guidelines: Subject + Solutions
Ask narrators to discuss a particular problem and offer a solution that parents and children can use immediately.

Presenter: Opening comments:

The diet of sedentary children is the same as that of sedentary adults. Adults, who adapt a sedentary lifestyle, generally do not teach their children to lead an active lifestyle. The children are likely to follow in the parents' footsteps. It is easy for children to become accustomed to high calorie snacks containing high fat and sugar instead of fruit, sandwiches, or other healthy foods because snacks with fat and sugar taste much better. When kids eat snacks between meals, they get all of the calories they need before dinner. If they consume all of the calories they need in snacks, the calories in the healthy food they eat will be stored as fat.

The best way to help children with weight problems is prevention and education. Don't let children have excessive amounts of junk food and sugar, and keep them involved in physical activities. Make sure their fun activities are related to exercise rather than allowing them to sit in front of a television or computer. Also, teach them about nutrition.

Note: While writing this book, I noticed many proud parents giving their three- and four-year-old children ice cream cones so big the children could hardly hold them with their little hands. I have noticed the same thing when parents give their children sodas and candy bars. When I see things like this, I think, "If they only knew!"

Use the following topics for research and planning purposes:
Who is responsible for your child's health?
Take the first step in managing your children's diet and food choices.

Sometimes the parent has to be the bad guy and make the tough decision.

Learn how to say no-thank-you to sweets and excess fats.

What works in maintaining good health? What doesn't work?

Negative Food Choices

Examples of Failure Regarding Negative food Choices

Positive Food Choices

Example of Success Regarding Positive Food Choices

How to stay on course after getting started

How to seek professional help

Join a support group

Exercise a minimum of twenty minutes each day

Presenter: Closing comments:

* What can overweight children expect as they get older if we don't take care of them now?

Killing Children with Kindness (KCK)

Help Our Children Manage their Health for the Future

Workshop #2, Topics for Discussion

Presenter 1:

* Diet and diet programs, how to make them work for your children and yourself.
* Fitness, and good health, how are they related
* Exercise: How to get started?

Presenter 2:

* Food facts as related to allergies, illnesses, and behavior
* How to make good food choices
* Two stories of success

Presenter 3: (An Overweight) A child may give this presentation.

* Hard facts about what to do to prevent obesity
* If your child is this age, weight, and height, what should you do to help the child maintain a healthy weigh and healthy lifestyle?
* Mom, it's your responsibility to make the hard decisions for your children. Make healthy choices for them. Don't be a pushover!

CHAPTER TWENTY-SEVEN

Guidelines for the Facilitator

Interviewing Children for a Video Presentation

THE GOALS OF an interview should be to give the workshop participants an up close and personal look at overweight children. This will let the people in the group get to know some overweight children and learn how they feel about being overweight. These children feel hurt when people are staring, teasing, or talking behind their back. Also, the audience should learn that being overweight is generally not the child's fault. It is the parent's fault when a child is overweight.

Suggested Starter:

* Hello Johnny, My name is Walter and we are making a video about children who are overweight. We want to show people that you are just like everyone else. I want to be able to show people that you are just a regular guy.
* I want you to do most of the talking. So I'm going to asking you some questions and give you a chance to tell people what you think.

1. First, introduce yourself and tell everyone what you enjoying doing for fun such as watching television, playing video games, going to movies, and other things like that.
2. Tell them what you like about school and what you would like to do when you grow up: doctor, lawyer, dentist, teacher, fireman, or police officer.
3. Is being overweight a problem for you? If so, how does being overweight bother you?
4. Do you think other people have problems with you being overweight?
5. How do you think you got to be overweight in the first place?
6. If you could give a message to other young children that would help keep them from getting overweight, what would you tell them?
7. If you could lose all of your excess weight down to your correct size, what would you do to keep the weight off?

Topic Starter:

Healthy Food Choices

When making healthy food choices, emphasis should be placed on choosing a variety of fruits and dark green leafy vegetables as well as bright-colored vegetables that are loaded with antioxidants and fiber. In addition, only complex carbohydrates are found in grain products and vegetables prepared without added sugar. The American Dietary Guidelines recommend eating at least half your grains as whole grains, which is at least 3 servings of whole grains a day. While on a diet, you may double this amount of whole grain in bread to lose weight.

According to a study published in the Archives of Internal Medicine, eating foods high in complex carbohydrates and low in fat can promote weight loss even without exercise.

The energy providing nutrients such as fat, carbohydrates, and protein, are used in proportion to each other in the body.

Therefore, basing a diet on any one food probably will not work simply because food should be used in balanced portions and variety.

The key to a healthy lifestyle starts with what you put in your mouth. It is as simple as that. This would include fruits, vegetables, meat, and fish. Too much fat causes you to gain weight just as too much protein and too much carbohydrate will cause you to gain. All three can make you fat if you eat too much of them.

If you currently drink soft drinks, it is imperative that you give up soft drinks first, because they are the worst sources of added sugars in the American diet.

Statistics and Facts

You may verify and update statistics on the Internet before using them:

Overweight is the excess amount of body weight that includes muscle, bone, fat, and water.

Obesity is the excess accumulation of body fat. One can be overweight without being obese: a body builder who has a lot of muscle, for example. However, for practical purposes, most people who are overweight are also obese.

Doctors and scientists generally agree that men with more than 25 percent body fat and women with more than 30 percent body fat are obese.

When a man's BMI is over 27.8, or woman's exceeds 27.3, that person is considered overweight. The degree of obesity associated with a particular BMI ranges from mild obesity at a BMI near 27, moderate obesity at 30, severe obesity at 35, to very severe obesity at 40 or greater. An estimated 41 percent of the population has a BMI greater than 25.

The number of overweight Americans increased from 25 to 33 percent between 1980 and 1991.

The survey also shows that minority populations, specifically minority women, are disproportionately affected: approximately 50 percent of African American and Mexican American women are overweight.

By a similar definition, more than one in five children and adolescents aged six through seventeen are also overweight.

Overweight and obesity is a known risk factor for diabetes, heart disease, high blood pressure, gallbladder disease, arthritis, breathing problems, and some forms of cancer.

Total number of overweight adults: (twenty through seventy-four years old) approximately one-third or 58 million Americans. (Numbers derived from NHANES III, 1988-91, which defines overweight as a BMI value of 27.3 percent or more for women and 27.8 percent or more for men)

* Overweight adult females (20-74 years old): 32 million (1990)
* Overweight adult males (20-74 years old): 26 million (1990)
* Total number of overweight youths: 6 through 17 years old approximately 11 percent or 4.7 million children

Other Overweight/Obesity-Related Statistics

* The number of extra calories a person must eat to gain a pound or burn to lose a pound:
  3,500 calories
* The percentage of adult American women trying to lose weight at any given time:
  33 to 40 percent
* The percentage of adult American men trying to lose weight at any given time:
  20 to 24 percent
* The average number of calories a person burns eating:
  .023 kcal per minute/per kilogram of body weight
* The annual number of deaths attributable to poor diet and inactivity:
  300,000 deaths

* Nearly 70 percent of the diagnosed cases of cardiovascular disease are related to obesity.
* Obesity accounts for $22.2 billion, or 19 percent, of the total cost of heart disease.

Obesity more than doubles one's chances of developing high blood pressure, which affects approximately 26 percent of obese American men and women. The annual cost of obesity-related high blood pressure is close to $1.5 billion dollars.

Almost half of breast cancer cases are diagnosed among obese women; an estimated 42 percent of colon cancer cases are diagnosed among obese individuals. Obesity-related breast cancer and colon cancer account for 2.5 percent of the total costs of cancer, or $1.9 billion dollars annually.

Americans spend an additional $33 billion dollars annually on weight-reduction products and services, including diet foods, products, and programs.

Globally, there are more than 1 billion overweight adults, at least 300 million of them obese.

Obesity and overweight pose a major risk for chronic diseases, including type-2 diabetes, cardiovascular disease, hypertension, stroke, and certain forms of cancer.

The key causes are increased consumption of energy-dense foods high in saturated fats and sugars, and reduced physical activity.

Things to Remember

1. Go on the Skip A Day Diet and stay on it. The diet will keep you from gaining weight while you condition your body until it can start burning fat.
2. Review the exercises and choose the ones that you can do safely. When you get started, increase the intensity, and duration of your exercises until you can stay active for up to one hour every other day.

3. If you are over fifty, do a twenty-minute session of light exercise when you get up in the morning and at night before you go to bed. Also, do a few exercises throughout the day to stay active.
4. Continue to diet, exercise, and practice sedentary avoidance until you reach your target weight. When you reach your target weight, go on a maintenance program to stay in shape.
5. Drink water

Visit the Skip A Day Diet Club Online

www.skipaday.com

Author's Insight

Developing the Skip A Day Diet Program has been a challenging task. Before I started working on it, I tried all of the traditional diets:

Very low carb diet
Very high carb diet
High protein diet
Very low fat diet
Moderately fat diet
Balanced diet

At times I would think "Nothing is going to work for me" because my body must be conforming to the set-point theory, which says that once your body reaches a certain weight, it becomes set at that new weight. The new weight would then be the acceptable weight that the body tries to maintain.

Besides being overweight, at times I had terrible back pain and my doctor would tell me that my cholesterol and blood pressure were up and that something bad was going to happen if I did not get my weight down. That would cause me to work at trying to lose weight again.

After experimenting with different diets, I decided to develop a new diet. My goal was to try and figure out how to improve on a diet that has proven itself through the years. Experts say that the balanced diet works, so I asked myself the question, Why should I reinvent the wheel if there is a diet that already works for everyone? I tried the balanced concept for a while, but it did not work very well. However, I did learn much valuable information while doing dieting research:

A diet unbalanced on the side of weight-gain will allow you to gain weight

A balanced diet will let you keep your present weight.

A diet unbalanced on the side of weight-loss will allow you to lose weight

Armed with this new information, I started working on a new diet, which would be unbalanced on the side of a weight loss. From that point on it should have been easy but, it took another seven years to completely develop and test this new diet program.

At first the new diet was called the "All Day Diet." During that phase of the research, I would skip both breakfast and lunch and eat one large meal at dinnertime. I lost about ten pounds on that version of the diet, but I had problems staying on it. At the time I was also on a rigorous exercise program, which (I found out later) added to the problem. I couldn't sustain both the diet and exercise over a long period of time because the calorie consumption was too low for the amount of exercise I was doing. I would either hurt myself from over exercising, or I would simply burnout from the diet and exercises. The process took on a pattern. I would stop dieting and exercising, get out of shape, and gain a few pounds. Then I would start back dieting and exercising again. This happened over and over for quite a number of years. I needed a diet/exercise program that I could stay on and lose weight. That is when I started testing the Skip A Day

Diet and conducting research to help put it together along with a low intensity exercise plan.

I thought that if I could skip two meals a day on the All Day Diet, why not skip all three meals one day and eat the next day? This version of the diet was better, but after a while I started to have problems with it. One of the problems was that I felt that I had to eat enough on eat-day to make up for the day I skipped. So I ate more than was necessary on eat-day.

I had no trouble skipping meals on diet days because I could get through the day just knowing that I could eat whatever I wanted the next day. However, it was difficult to eat even a small snack without triggering my appetite. When that happened, I would eat more than I should and whatever I wanted. I just knew that if I could cut back two meals a day, the fat would start flying off, but that did not happen.

At the time I was experimenting with a lot of different diet/exercise combinations, so when something caused me to lose a few pounds, I would focus on what I thought caused the weight loss. The pattern kept coming back. With food, when I ate plain-food meals too long, I would get bored with them. With exercise, when I over-exercised, I would burnout.

I thought that whatever finally worked for me would no doubt work for others. That's when I started writing this book. My goal was to come up with a diet that works and to share it with others as soon as possible. However, it took much longer than I expected to develop the diet and write the book.

The only thing that finally worked well for me was the volume component of the diet. It allowed me to eat a wide variety of delicious foods and fill my stomach to capacity with a staple that kept me full. In my search for a suitable staple, I tried several combinations with: vegetables, legumes, brown rice, and potatoes. After a while I started to experiment with different breads. I soon found that bread works the way I wanted a staple to work. It filled me up without a lot of extra calories.

The breads that I like include multi-grain, whole grain, and whole wheat bread. In order to stay with the skip a day concept, I would eat bread, vegetables, poultry, meat, and fish on eat days and use only breads, vegetables, and spreads on diet-day. This worked well until I started using too many and too much spread on the bread. When I counted up the calories, I found that I was consuming too much fat in the delicious spreads. Then I had to cut back on the best spreads and use more of the high volume, low calorie spreads such as a veggie spread that I made my self.

After a while I started to use mostly veggie spreads along with different toppings on the veggie spread and other low fat spreads on the bread. By using more vegetables and spreads with less oils and fats, I cut my calorie consumption down to about 1,200 on eat-day and 600 hundred on diet-day. This allowed me to start to lose weight consistently. That is when I felt as though I had finally taken control over my body.

I believe that I was able to adjust to the diet because of the variety of breads, vegetables, meats, and spreads I had every day. Even though I eat mostly bread with my meals, I was able to continue on the diet and lose weight.

At one point I became comfortable eating nothing at all on diet-day. Then I read a report that suggested that I might not be getting enough fat in my meals. That is when I started to eat a handful of nuts on eat-day. I also included more fish in my meals. This gave me the fats and oils I needed. I probably was consuming enough fat without the nuts and extra fish, but I adding them anyway just to be safe.

Researchers have shown over and over that people who follow a diet low in fat and high in fiber lose weight. This is an established fact. However, the problem with following those simple instructions was "How to put together a diet that could be followed day after day." The food had to taste good. The Skip A Day Diet has evolved to a point where it works well for me and the other people who have tried it, and the food tastes great. Will it work for everyone? That has to be determined from trials and research. In the meantime, I believe that it will work for most of the people who need to lose weight, and it can be done without a lot of exercise.

Now that I look back at the development process, all of the time spent trying the various diets was only part of the research because nothing actually worked until I fully developed the Skip A Day diet and lost weight with it.

I gained a lot of knowledge about dieting while conducting research for this program, but it all comes down to this: The Skip A Day Diet, whole grain breads, vegetables without added fats, spreads without added fats, lean meat with all of the fat and skin removed, nuts, fish, and the Upside Down Quarter all come together to make the weight-loss program work.

CHAPTER TWENTY-EIGHT

So why is it so hard to lose weight?

THE SHORT ANSWER is "Because we overeat!" It seems that we not only overeat, but we overeat to the extreme. A certain overweight, sedentary man may only need about 1,600 calories a day, but some days he may consume over 3,000. When he eats 3,000 calories, his body may get to process, store, and use only 2,100 calories of the food he consumes that day. This means that he will gain only 500 of the extra 1400 calories as excess weight. Knowing this, we can say that he has the capacity to absorb 500 extra calories a day and gain a pound a week.

The extra, 900 calories that were not used, will pass through the system as waste. When he eats three meals a day, the same thing happens every day. The body will not have had time to extract all the nutrients from the food before new food comes through and pushes it out of the system. This means that he will be wasting 900 calories in nutrient rich poop every day. He has the potential to continue to gain about one pound a week as long as his meals are at or above 2,100 calories per day.

When he becomes obese, and gets a life threatening disease such diabetes, his doctor may encourage him to go on a diet. Out of fear, he may cut food consumption down to 2,100 calories a day and start walking for exercise. After a few weeks, he sees no changes because his body will still be absorbing 500 extra calories each day. He may even gain a couple of pounds and quit dieting and exercising out of frustration.

This is why ordinary diets don't work. When he cuts only 900 calories from his diet, he will not even scratch the surface because he only cut the calories his body cannot take in. He would have to cut calorie consumption down to 1,600 a day just to keep from gaining weight. Then he would have to cut another 500 calories just to see a significant weight loss over period of time. This would put him down to 1,100 calories a day. It is a viscous cycle. He will never win at the losing game because the odds are stacked against him especially if he doesn't know what's going on with his body. He is not the only one going through this. Few people will be willing to accept the idea that eating only one balanced meal a day is better for them. It is inconceivable that they should skip a day of eating regular meals just to lose weight, even if it means saving their lives.

People overeat because they have a strong appetite. They have no idea that they can control the monster. We normally establish our appetite while we are young and active. Everyone knows it by heart: Eat three meals a day with a small breakfast, a medium sized lunch, and a large dinner. If we miss one of these meals, the chemicals that control our appetite, will make us feel like we are going to die from starvation. The empty feeling is real. The pain and headaches are real. And the many other symptoms are real. You have no way of knowing that if you start skipping one day of eating, the symptoms will begin to go away and disappear in a few days.

Obviously, not everyone has the same problem with appetite control. If that were the case, all of us in the United States would be overweight. One possible reason more of us are not over weight is because our bodies do not have the ability to process and take in more calories than we need each day. If a twenty-four year old woman has high metabolism, and her body can process and keep only 2,100 calories a day; she might be able to eat 3,000 calories a day and never gain a pound because her body will not be storing extra calories. The extra 900 calories would go right through her and come out as waste. However, that is not the case with everyone.

Let's take a look at another active 25-year-old female who has high metabolism and only needs 1,600 calories per day. She also has the capacity to take in an extra 500 calories per day. Her daily activities include selling real estate, jogging, and walking with her dog in the evenings. Her weekend activities include an aerobics class on Saturday and a tennis match on Sunday. She too can consume 3,000 calories a day and not gain weight because she burns off the extra 500 calories her body takes in. The unused 400 calories left over will be taken away with waste. As long as she is active, there is no problem. But when she gets married, things begin to change.

For a while, things will stay the same except that her clothes may get a little tight, but that is okay; what's wrong with a few extra pounds? However, when she gets pregnant everything changes. While she is pregnant she may gain an extra ten pounds. After all, she has to eat for two. She will be able to burn off the extra fat in no time. At least that is what she thinks.

This is what really happens. During the nine months of pregnancy she got out of shape and is not as physically fit as she was before. She no longer has the luxury of going out jogging and walking the dog every day. She is too busy caring for the child, cooking, and cleaning the house.

She realizes that she has to cut calories because she wants to lose the extra fat. The sweets are the first thing to go, but they might be replaced with fast food. Who has time to manage a career, take care of a child, and cook? This sets the stage.

Since she has been programmed to eat three meals a day, and that programming is reinforced with chemical reactions in the body, she thinks that she has no other choice. So, she continues to eat three meals a day that ad up to over 2,100 calories a day. This caused the excess weight to keep creeping on the waistline and hips. She can't understand it. She is eating far less than she was eating before she got pregnant. What's wrong?

By not selling real estate, jogging, taking daily walks with her dog, and working out on the weekend, she is not burning off the extra

500 calories that her body takes in each day. She may gain only one or two pounds a month but it adds up after a while. Now she is caught up in the cycle that leads to obesity.

What can she do before it gets to this point? The first thing she should do is realize, that there is no natural law that says she has to eat three meals a day. She can consume one well, balanced meal a day and remain healthy. As a matter of fact, the human body has been designed by nature; to handle one large meal a day better than it can handle three regular meals a day. Here is why.

First of all, the meal can be consumed over a period of three hours. It can start at five o'clock in the evening and end at eight o'clock at night. When someone consumes a large meal that contains a variety of fats, proteins, and complex carbohydrates, the body releases digestive juices into the stomach. The juices will liquefy the food and prepares it for digestion. To aid with digestion, the stomach muscles will relax and allow the stomach to expand so that more of the food will be exposed to the digestive juices inside the stomach. This starts the digestion process, which can take up to twelve hours especially for fats, meats, protein, and milk products.

Let's assume that this woman had her last snack of the day at just before bedtime or around 10 P.M. Since the entire meal can take up to twelve hours to completely digest, she will have undigested food in her stomach when she gets up in the morning.

Remember that while she was physically active during the day, digestion stopped. This means that most digestion will take place while she is resting or sleeping. After digestion in the stomach takes place, the food moves into the small intestines where the majority of the nutrients are absorbed and stored until it is either used as energy or stored as fat. Food moving into the small intestines adds to the stomach's swelling and is part of the natural digestion cycle.

It is much easier on the body if digestion takes place only once in twenty-four hours. By eating only one meal a day the human body conforms to this natural cycle. By eating three meals a day, it upsets the natural cycle. Here is what can happen when the cycle is upset.

When you get up in the morning, your stomach, small intestines, and colon will be still full of food from the previous day. Since you will be hungry in the morning, you will eat breakfast having the regular: toast, two eggs, a glass of milk, and a glass of juice. The body releases fluids into the stomach and the stomach expands to aid in digestion. This starts the twelve-hour digestion process. Some people call this bloating and may feel uncomfortable the rest of the day. Bloating reaches its peak about five hours after the digestion process starts. Also, since you will be active throughout the day, digestion will be slower. In any case the breakfast meal will still be in your stomach at lunchtime.

At lunchtime you decide to have a regular lunch, which consists of a green salad, and a club sandwich, a slice of pie, and glass of sweet tea. New food going into the stomach interrupts the digestion process that was started by breakfast. Since this lunch meal is larger than the breakfast meal, digestion starts over. Juices are released into the stomach to breakdown the food for digestion. Since it takes a lot of energy to process your food, you may begin the feel tired and weak. You might even feel a little sick and get an upset stomach as the food backs up in the stomach.

By dinnertime all of the discomfort will have passed and you have a hardy appetite again. This is good because now you feel like enjoying a good hardy dinner. After all, this is normally the largest meal of the day. It has been a long day and you don't feel like cooking dinner, so it is fast food for the family. Dad and the children want pizza, but you want something that's easier to digest, so you compromise and order pizza for them and a green salad for yourself. A slice of pizza, green salad, desert, and a diet soda will be a good healthy meal. After all, you are watching your weight.

What a day this has been. The trouble started with that bloated feeling after lunch. Then you got sick in the afternoon. Now, here it is 11 o'clock at night and you're sitting up in bed with heartburn. All of your food is backing up again. Lately, this is getting to be a chronic condition. Thank goodness for antacids. When will this vicious cycle end?

Read between the lines: Your stomach is always full. Digestion gets interrupted every day. You are always tired and weak. Acid reflux is killing you. You are constantly gaining weight. You have severe back pain. You don't have time to exercise. You don't like exercise. You feel like falling asleep after lunch. Your husband is getting fat. Your kids are getting fat. Your dog is getting fat, and your cat is getting fat. Go figure!

Try this: one meal a day, one digestion cycle a day, one expenditure of energy per day for digestion, and a brief nap after dinner equals a good night's sleep.

So, the next time you find yourself standing in front of the refrigerator with the door open, dismiss it by saying Oh, "I just ate yesterday. It's just the ghrelin spiking."

References

Berlin, J.A., and G.A. Colditz. "A meta-analysis of physical activity in the prevention of coronary heart disease." *Am J Epidemiol* 132 (1990): 639-46.

Blair, S.N., H.W. Kohl, R.S. Paffenbarger, Jr, D.G. Clark, K.H. Cooper, and L.W. Gibbons. "Physical fitness and all-cause mortality: a prospective study of healthy men and women." *JAMA* 262 (1989): 2395-401.

Fletcher, G.F., S.N. Blair, and J. Blumenthal, et al. "Statement on exercise—benefits and recommendations for physical activity programs for all Americans: a statement for health professionals by the Committee on Exercise and Cardiac Rehabilitation of the Council on Clinical Cardiology." *American Heart Association* 86 (Circulation 1992): 340-4.

Kluger, Jeffrey. "The Science of Appetite," Special Health Report. *Time Magazine*. The series runs through pages 49-82.

Paffenbarger Jr., R. S., R. T. Hyde, A. L. Wing, I. M. Lee, D. L. Jung, and J.B. Kampert. "The association of changes in physical-activity level and other lifestyle characteristics with mortality among men." *N Engl J Med* 328 (1993): 538-45.

Powell, K.E., P. D. Thompson, C. J. Caspersen, and J. S. Kendrick. "Physical activity and the incidence of coronary heart disease." *Annu Rev Public Health* 8 (1987): 253-87.

US Department of Health and Human Services, Public Health Service, "Healthy people 2000: national health promotion and disease prevention objectives—full report, with commentary." Washington, DC, 1991. *DHHS publication no. (PHS)* 91-50212.

Siegel, P. Z., R. M. Brackbill, and E. L. Frazier, et al. *Behavioral Risk Factor Surveillance* 40 (1986-1990.MMWR 1991; no. SS-4): 1-23.

Shah, B.V., "SESUDAAN: standard errors program for computing of standardized rates from sample survey data." Research Triangle Park, North Carolina: Research Triangle Institute, 1981.

More References

American College of Sports Medicine, *ACSM's Guidelines for Exercise Testing and Prescription*, ed 5, Baltimore, Williams & Wilkins, 1995.

Andersen, R. E., S. N. Blair, and L. J. Cheskin, et al. "Encouraging patients to become more physically active: the physician's role." *Ann Intern Med* 127 (1997): (5) 395-400.

Andersen, R. E., C. J. Crespo, and S. J. Bartlett, et al. "Relationship of physical activity and television watching with body weight and level of fatness among children: results from the Third National Health and Nutrition Examination Survey." *JAMA* 279 (1998): (12) 938-942.

Andersen, R.E., "Physiology of obesity in," ed. R.T. Cotton, Lifestyle and Weight Management Consultant Manual. San Diego, *American Council on Exercise.* (1996): 95-118.

Andersen, R.E., T. A. Wadden, and S. J. Bartlett, et al. "Effects of lifestyle activity vs. structured aerobic exercise in obese women: a randomized trial." *JAMA* 281 (1999): (4) 335-340.

Ballor, D.L., and E. T. Poehlman. "A meta-analysis of the effects of exercise and/or dietary restriction on resting metabolic rate." *Eur J Appl Physiol* 71 (1995): (6):535-542.

Blair, S.N. "1993 C.H. McCloy Research Lecture: physical activity, physical fitness, and health." *Res Q Exerc Sport* 64 (1993): (4):365-376.

Brownell, K. D. "Exercise in the treatment of obesity," Edited by K. D. Brownell and C. G. Fairburn. *Eating Disorders and Obesity: A Comprehensive Handbook*. New York City, Guilford Press, (1995): 473-478.

Crespo, C. J., R. E. Andersen, and M. Pratt, et al. "Obesity and its relation to physical activity and television watching among US children." *Med Sci Sports Exerc* 30 (1998): (5 suppl) S80.

Crespo, C. J. and J. D. Wright. "Prevalence of overweight among active and inactive US adults from the Third National Health and Nutrition Examination Survey." *Med Sci Sports Exerc* 27 (1995): (5 suppl) S73.

DeBusk, R. F., U. Stenestrand, and M. Sheehan, et al. "Training effects of long versus short bouts of exercise in healthy subjects." *Am J Cardio* l65 (1990): (15) 1010-1013.

Dunn, A. L., B. H. Marcus, and J. B. Kampert, et al. "Comparison of lifestyle and structured interventions to increase physical activity and cardiorespiratory fitness: a randomized trial. *JAMA* 281 (1999): (4) 327-334.

Fletcher, G. F, G. Balady, and S. N. Blair, et al. "Statement on exercise: benefits and recommendations for physical activity programs for all Americans: a statement for health professionals by the Committee on Exercise and Cardiac Rehabilitation of the Council on Clinical Cardiology." *American Heart Association.* Circulation 94 (1996): (4) 857-862.

Grilo, C. M., K. D. Brownell, and A. J. Stunkard. "The metabolic and psychological importance of exercise in weight control." Edited by A.J. Stunkard and T. A.Wadden. *Obesity: Theory and Therapy.* New York City, Raven Press, (1993): 253-273.

Jakicic, J. M., R. R. Wing, and B. A. Butler, et al. "Prescribing exercise in multiple short bouts versus one continuous bout: effects on adherence, cardiorespiratory fitness, and weight loss in overweight women." *Int J Obes Relat Metab Disord* 19 (1995): (12) 893-901.

Jakicic, J. M. and R. R.Wing. "Strategies to improve exercise adherence: effect of short-bouts versus long-bouts of exercise." *Med Sci Sports Exerc* 29 (1997): (5 suppl) S42.

Kayman, S, W. Bruvold, and J. S. Stern. "Maintenance and relapse after weight loss in women: behavioral aspects." *Am J Clin Nutr* 52 (1990): (5) 800-807.

King, A.C. and D. L. Tribble. "The role of exercise in weight regulation in nonathletes." *Sports Med* 11 (1991): (5) 331-349.

Kuczmarski, R. J., M. D. Carroll, and K. M. Flegal, et al. "Varying body mass index cutoff points to describe overweight prevalence among US adults." *NHANES III (1988 to 1994).* Obes Res 5 1997: (6) 542-548.

Lee, C. D., S. N. Blair, A. S. Jackson. "Cardiorespiratory fitness, body composition, and all-cause and cardiovascular disease mortality in men." *Am J Clin Nutr* 69 (1999): (3) 373-380.

Melby, C., C. Scholl, and G. Edwards, et al. "Effect of acute resistance exercise on postexercise energy expenditure and resting metabolic rate." *J Appl Physiol* 75 (1993): (4) 1847-1853.

National Institutes of Health: "Physical activity and cardiovascular health: NIH Consensus Development Panel on Physical Activity and Cardiovascular Health." *JAMA* 276 (1996): (3) 241-246.

Pate, R. R., M. Pratt, and S. N. Blair, et al. "Physical activity and public health: a recommendation from the Centers for Disease Control and Prevention and the American College of Sports Medicine." *JAMA* 273 (1995): (5) 402-407.

Poehlman, E. T. "A review: exercise and its influence on resting energy metabolism in man." *Med Sci Sports Exerc* 21 (1989): (5) 515-525.

Poehlman, E. T., M. J. Toth, and P. A. Ades, et al. "Gender differences in resting metabolic rate and noradrenalin kinetics in older individuals." *Eur J Clin Invest* 27 (1997): (1) 23-28.

Pollock, M. L., G. A. Gaesser, and J. D. Butcher, et al. "The recommended quantity and quality of exercise for developing and maintaining cardiorespiratory and muscular fitness, and flexibility in healthy adults." *Med Sci Sports Exerc* 30 (1998): (6) 975-991.

Prentice, A. M. and S. A. Jebb. "Obesity in Britain: gluttony or sloth?" *BMJ* 311 (1995): (7002) 437-439.

U.S. Department of Health and Human Services. "Physical Activity and Health: A Report of the Surgeon General, Atlanta, DHHS, Centers for Disease Control and Prevention." National Center for Chronic Disease Prevention and Health Promotion, 1996.

Vidal-Puig, A., G. Solanes, and D. Grujic, et al. "UCP3: an uncoupling protein homologue expressed preferentially and abundantly in skeletal muscle and brown adipose tissue." *Biochem Biophys Res Commun* 235 (1997): (1) 79-82.

*Reference Note: A paper by Browning, CU-Boulder integrative physiology Associate Professor Rodger Kram and undergraduates Emily Baker and Jessica Herron was presented at the June 2005 meeting of the American College of Sports Medicine meeting in Nashville and published recently in the journal, "Obesity Research." Article Date: 16 Jun 05.www.medicalnewstoday.com. Also confirmed for several other sources.

www.ingramcontent.com/pod-product-compliance
Lightning Source LLC
Chambersburg PA
CBHW051419280526
45785CB00003B/1079